MW01247521

SUBTLE
STROKE

SUBTLE STROKE

The SOFT, SUBTLE, SPIRITUAL
awakening of stroke recovery . . .

By Rachel Jarmusz

gatekeeper press

Subtle Stroke:
The Soft, Subtle, Spiritual Awakening of Stroke Recovery

Published by Gatekeeper Press
7853 Gunn Hwy., Suite 209
Tampa, FL 33626
www.GatekeeperPress.com

Yoga is not a substitute for medical attention, examination, diagnosis or treatment. I am not a doctor, nor a yoga therapist. I cannot say yoga is therapy or will heal any medical condition. As a yoga practitioner you must affirm by participating in any yoga practice, I am assuming all risk and have gotten the approval of my doctors, if necessary.

Back Cover Image by Octavia Morgan, Level 3 / Intermediate Senior 1 Certified Iyengar Yoga Teacher at Yoga Shala in Boulder, CO.
Illustrations by Katelyn Woodruff

ISBN (paperback): 9781662949463
eISBN: 9781662949470

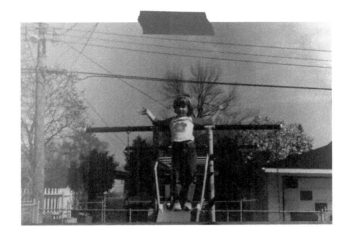

For her.

five-year-old Rachel, fearless and full of life.

TABLE OF CONTENTS

A PLAY ON WORDS

According to the CDC, a *stroke* occurs when something blocks blood supply to the brain or when a blood vessel in the brain bursts. In either case, parts of the brain become damaged or die, often causing long-term disability or death.

In commonplace language a stroke, as defined by *Webster's*, is the act of hitting or striking or a mark made by a pen, pencil, or paintbrush. The medical community says it's something that causes a loss of blood flow to the brain; a stroke, a blow or strike to the brain. Therefore, if a stroke is a brain injury, what then strikes the brain? The medical community is saying that something you cannot see and cannot always explain hits or strikes you on the top of your head and causes loss of blood flow to the brain in various ways. It's an interesting choice of words, if you ask me.

There are as many strokes as people on this planet, just as unique and powerful each time, like a lightning bolt. No one stroke can be compared to another and every recovery process is different, yet somehow we begin to uncover themes.

Well, they are saying it without saying it. It is the unseen world, dare I say *Energy*. Something unexplainable strikes the head, causing a complete shift in reality. It often causes huge shifts in personality, like the woman who had a stroke and woke up with a British accent. Foreign accent syndrome happens in about every 2 out of 10 strokes (according to WebMD).

Ongoing abuse, let's say as a child, such as physical, sexual, emotional, or mental can cause lesions on the brain similar to a stroke. Outside of stroke survivors, many people are experiencing ongoing brain trauma that influences behavior patterns and emotions. The principles in this book can be applied to any human being. Whether you yourself had a stroke, you are a loved one of a stroke survivor, caregiver, or any trauma survivor out there. I chose to write about stroke because I was fortunate to gain this experience.

If you asked me how to define a stroke, I would say it was an alteration in brain tissue for a variety of reasons that allows the brain an opportunity to access new pathways and create new nerve endings, ultimately ending up with heightened awareness, or the catalyst for a spiritual awakening—a new conscious stream that replaces an old, more rigid way of being. An opportunity, really, like installing a portal to a higher-conscious stream. I believe a stroke cracks open the third eye. Severe brain trauma in general allows a deeper connection to the divine source of energy within, giving direct access to the "subtle body."

Our thoughts or our conscious stream are a portal for the divine. There are many of these in our human body—the mind, the heart, and the feet being just a basic few of these channels or pathways, portals to the divine—places we can access universal consciousness, god or creator energy center, source, Krishna, Jesus Christ (Christ consciousness), whatever title you like. You literally are the universe in motion, divine energy in physical form.

I have heard many medical professionals and stroke survivors themselves reference a stroke as a brain "attack." Right away, this terminology puts us at war with our body. Attack literally means aggressive action. Words are powerful. Why not reframe the view of a stroke as a brain "opportunity" rather than an "attack"? Well, because of the hold the pharmaceutical companies have on doctors and rehab centers, creating dependent customers as well as the limited knowledge base within the medical education system about the body and energy. It's as if they were ignoring a whole set of tools with bias. Not educating these medical professionals properly is malpractice, in my opinion.

Why not reframe stroke, and the education these stroke professionals receive, widen their scope? This is the question that inspired me to write this book. I had my stroke in 2009, a thromboembolic (blood clot) stroke, or a striatocapsular stroke with Wallerian degeneration, on 6/12/2009.

According to Radiopedia, "A striatocapsular infarct, also known as a basal ganglionic capsular infarct, is an infarct involving the caudate nucleus, putamen, and the internal capsule without any involvement of the cortex, usually caused by a cerebral artery occlusion."

It goes on to say basal ganglia are "a group of gray matter nuclei in the deep aspects of the brain interconnected to the brainstem, cerebral cortex and thalami."

So it's a deep stroke, deep inside the nucleus of brain cells, the center of a cell.

My stroke was deep within the grey matter of my brain, what they called an ischemic event (inadequate supply of blood, in this case to the brain). According to the *Oxford Dictionary*, ischemia is a Greek word meaning "stopping blood." Also, it could mean to hold back. My right carotid artery tore on a roller coaster and caused a clot to break off and travel to my brain, creating a lot of pressure within my head. The pain is something most stroke survivors never forget. The most intense pain anyone could ever experience, it really is the worst headache you've ever had. A migraine on crack.

By the grace of god and at the hands of a talented, brilliant female neurologist, my brain began to heal almost as quickly as it began to stroke out.

After my stroke, my rapid recovery seemed to amaze most doctors. I was in rehab for about thirty days and relearned life—eating, drinking, speaking, walking, dressing, showering. I rapidly came back to life and movement. My limbs still struggled to work as I desired. I needed ongoing therapy to continue to regain function of my body. For years I did everything the medical community suggested.

I saw some of the best physios and neurologists in the country. I always came up short, wondering what was really missing in my recovery. My MRI check-in a year later showed consistent Wallerian degeneration on my brain stem caused by a dissected carotid artery, affecting upper-left limb mobility—face, shoulder, hand, hip, and foot hemiparesis.

It would be hard to access this deep place within my brain.

Because of the location and size of my stroke, I am unlikely to regain use of my upper-left extremity, but more progress has been made from the moment my doctors told me I'd never get any relief in my elbow without surgery or Botox. I don't ever want another stroke survivor to feel like they are past the point of their own recovery.

Recovery is all about faith and grace.

Faith and grace: Two spiritual, mental, and emotional aspects of healing our modern medical community completely ignores. To me, my therapy always felt incomplete. It appeared there was one recovery funnel all stroke survivors went through. Recovery was not individualized or expansive. To me it felt limiting and very basic. I'm appreciative of many of the doctors, PTs, and OTs I had, but I was always left asking where's the rest?

Subtlety was missing. I couldn't put a finger on the word back then, but it is subtle. There is only gross matter—a physical, muscular approach to stroke recovery being shoved down all stroke survivors' throats—and many are simply denied access to basic rehabilitation to begin with, while most of the recovery process is a part of the unseen world or this subtle body.

Let's switch gears to the title of this book: *Subtle Stroke*.

Subtle is a word meaning delicately complex and understated. I don't think there could be a better word to pair with a stroke. In this book, we unpack the delicate components of a stroke and the complex, subtle recovery process with a soft individualized approach.

Some have the standard signs—high blood pressure, overweight, and high cholesterol, but others go undiagnosed. A cryptogenic stroke is what it's called, and 1 in 3 ischemic strokes are cryptogenic. Mine was such.

The nervous system is a subtle network of more than 100 billion nerves firing throughout our day. I imagine our energy oozing out of our bodies, like a massive cloud of protection around us. We are never alone; we carry the universe within us. It's no wonder it's hard for the medical community to try and contain, let alone explain. It's not containable and somewhat hard to explain without sounding like a nut.

In spiritual texts, such as the Bhagavad Gita and Upanishads, the *subtle body* is referenced as a combination of the ego, mind, and intelligence controlling the physical body. It is neither the soul nor gross matter, but rather the in-between layers or sheaths.

Some might say the subtle body is otherwise known as the energetic body or pranic (breath) body wrapped by matter within the gross body. It does not house or protect the soul, rather it protects the conscious idea or understanding of the soul, because the soul really can't be contained, it oozes all around, it has no bounds. I believe the subtle body may rest within the complex layer of *fascia* deep within our body.

Fascia being this intricate delicate webbing of tissues, similar to sausage casing, holding all of our insides together.

As the Vedas explain, these sheaths or layers are known as Koshas, covering the conscious idea of the soul, like layers of an onion if you will. From outer to inner:

1. **Annamaya Kosha**: Food sheath
2. **Pranamaya Kosha**: Life force breath sheath
3. **Manomaya Kosha**: Mental sheath
4. **Vijnanamaya Kosha**: Wisdom sheath
5. **Anandamaya Kosha**: Bliss sheath

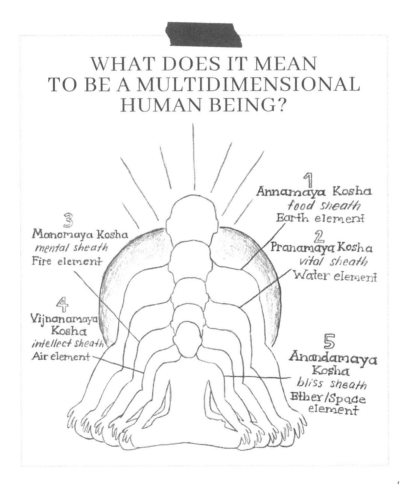

When it comes to yoga, tantra, Taoism, or Hinduism, any form of spirituality really, the subtle body is key to understanding the self.

Western medicine completely ignores these components of the WHOLE body.

Or as I emphasize, WHOLISTIC (I refuse to diminish the word to Holistic). That W matters.

Reminding folks that they are the WHOLE package. Everything inside.

Remember, we as humans are physical, spiritual, emotional, and mental beings all living under one roof, so to speak.

In Sanskrit, this subtle body is often referred to as a Linga Sharira or Astral body.

Sanskrit (meaning refined or perfected) is one of the oldest spoken languages of humans, and a good amount of our yoga language has roots in this beautiful language. All other languages stem from it. Many minimize it to the language of Hinduism or India, but it is far more than that. *Britannica* says, "an adorned, cultivated, purified, old Indo-Aryan language, composed in what is called Vedic Sankrit." The Vedic Documents represent the dialect then found in the northern midlands of the Indian Subcontinent, which scholars generally apply to 1500 BCE.

Have you ever wondered what our ancestors were talking about when they first realized they could verbally communicate with each other?

Some might say Sanskrit was delivered to humans by the sounds of each Chakra more than 3,500 years ago, beginning as just stringing syllables together to begin to construct words and language. (We discuss the chakras later in depth.)

Common Sanskrit yoga language includes:

- **Namaste** or Namaskar: has remained a common greeting in some Indian cultures, not always having to do with yoga. The word itself means hello, welcome, I bow to you, praise to you, I honor you, I see you. The word has many different translations.
- **Yoga:** Yuj, yoke, or union.
- **Ohm:**
  - Pronounced more like A-U-M
  - Represents the universal sound of the universe (NASA has a recording of this vibrational sound from space). The sound that unites us all, literally!
- **Hatha Yoga:** a term for a physical sequence of Asana designed to bring balance to the body, combining both strength and flexibility, yoga in the physical sense. The word Hatha means sun and moon.
- **Vinyasa:** a type of yoga in which the poses flow into one another using the breath. Meaning "linking movement to breath."
- **Yoga Nidra:** Yogic sleep. Typically, a meditation done lying down is designed to achieve ultimate relaxation between the sleep state and the conscious state. One hour of yoga nidra is equivalent to four hours of restful sleep.
- **Prana:** breath or life force energy.

As we learn more about the Astral plane and this universal cosmic energy, I believe more awareness of the human brain will occur, as the two are very much linked.

TYPES OF STROKES

There are three major types of strokes, and each is unique in its own way. I experienced an ischemic stroke. I say "experienced" rather than "suffered" because we need to change the language we use in the stroke community, eliminating words like "suffered" and "victim." Our words matter, and they can either empower us or disempower us.

Types of strokes, according to the American Stroke Association:

- **Ischemic:** blood vessels supplying blood to the brain become obstructed.
- **Hemorrhagic:** a weakened blood vessel rupture.
- **Tia:** mini stroke caused by a serious temporary blood clot.

> **Stroke is the fifth leading cause of death in the US.**
> **Stroke is the leading cause of disability in the US.**

One in four stroke survivors has a second stroke. That rate almost doubles the younger the age of the survivor.

According to the *Journal of the American Heart Association*, there are many conditions said to cause stroke, such as AFIB, PFO, Aortic Atheroma, and hypercoagulable states, just to name a few that are said to directly link to stroke.

Biology teaches us that blood is the vehicle oxygen uses to circulate through our body, so when the blood flow to the brain is compromised, literally every second matters until that blood flow and oxygen flow are restored to the brain. This is why knowing the warning signs can be very crucial. But often, no warning signs present; well, not in the way of Act Fast: Face, Arms, Speech, Time.

Also, if breathing exercises were administered in patients very quickly after the stroke itself, recovery rates would increase. I'm sure of that. No one should be permanently disabled from a stroke.

Stroke is in an interesting trend right now as the rate of stroke is nearly doubling each year, yet the age of average stroke is dropping. I forget where I read that, but it sure is an interesting trend.

Every stroke has varying degrees of severity, and some people recover more quickly, some take more time. I have been fortunate to be one of those slow, more subtle recoveries.

At first, it seemed quick. I was making gains, eating, talking, standing, but then I kind of hit a wall and to be honest, I don't know that I will ever be "fully" recovered. Plateaus, they say. I got so sick of this word that I choose "redirection" as a more suitable description.

I'm not even sure what that means. Plateaus are natural occurrences. They are beautiful and breathtaking in many ways. Yet many insurance companies deny therapy when patients hit this so-called plateau. Instead of simply switching up the therapy, they deny renewed scripts for ongoing therapy, leaving many frustrated and lonely at home.

But I know recovery from any severe trauma is a journey, not a destination. A marathon, not a sprint.

Some people look at me and are impressed with how far I have come, and some look and say I have so much farther to go.

I honor both opinions.

I try my best to neither look back nor forward but to be in the present moment. *The Power of Now* by Eckhart Tolle was the very first text I read on my teacher training journey. A great book to begin for those curious about embarking on a spiritual path.

"Now" or "Atha" is the first yoga sutra as well, this idea of being where you are fully and completely. Acceptance can be very hard for stroke survivors. I think it took me a good five years to accept that I didn't break a leg, and that rest and vitamins would not restore me to the person I once was. I was forever changed, so I began my journey of self-acceptance and self-love in this new body.

Looking at the *Yoga Sutras of Patanjali*, translation and commentary by Swami Satchidanada, we can see that the first few yoga Sutras (threads) are all about the brain, the mind, the thoughts, not the body or exercise:

- **SUTRA I.1** Now the exposition of yoga is being made.
- **SUTRA I.2** The restraint of the modifications of the mind-stuff is yoga.
- **SUTRA I. 3** The seer (self) abides in its own nature.

Okay, so I want to begin a yoga practice now. Where do I begin? The world would have you believe you need yoga pants and a cute yoga mat. Or you need to be fit and flexible to begin. These misconceptions keep many from receiving the benefits of yoga, this beautiful practice rooted in self-awareness and compassion. While goal-setting and using goals as a kind of compass can be helpful, I often try not to focus too much on specifics. I'd rather slowly welcome myself back into myself, staying in the present in each moment, just breathing.

A GOOD PLACE TO BEGIN: CREATE YOUR OWN PERSONAL GOALS.

What will your yoga do for you?

My Yoga Will:

1. ....
....
....

2. ....
....
....

3. ....
....
....

4. ....
....
....

As the Bhagavad Gita says, "Yoga is the journey of the self through the self."

No rush.

Welcome yourself home. Namaste.

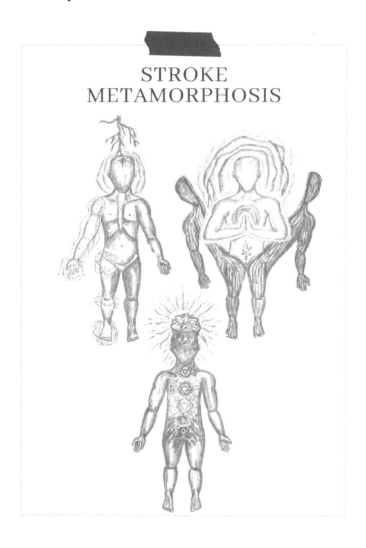

STROKE
METAMORPHOSIS

CHAPTER 1

LOVE

Love, in our culture, is often based on actions or an external circumstance. You behaved well, you dressed well, you got a good grade, you helped a neighbor—I love you so much!!

Withholding love was often a punishment. Financial security was often perceived as love for certain generations.

Love was and often is conditional. Love often has no physical displays, making that natural human need for touch and connection sparse.

Often, children come into this world choosing parents that may not be able to love them in the best ways. It is often a harsh realization that we choose our parents as we are coming into this life, for the soul's best advancement.

Growing up in my family was not always easy.

I can be mad at my family for the trauma I experienced as a young child and love them for doing their best at the same time.

I have gone through a full range of emotions when it comes to my parents.

My family has had its fair share of struggle and hardship; my parents have endured more trauma than I could ever imagine, and my siblings are both thriving despite many setbacks. They have always given me inspiration to pursue my dreams. For me though, I've always been a bit different. I always had a unique way of looking at the world, being the crazy, silly, messy-haired, mismatched-sock kind of weird kid. Quiet . . . always in my head. Always reading or giggling uncontrollably.

Following the standard path was never my thing. I really must work on maintaining positive thoughts and staying motivated, because I have always thought so deeply about things and since my stroke experience such extreme brain fog and exhaustion from things that used to appease me.

Brain fog is a cognitive impairment that can cause difficulty concentrating, dizziness, confusion, inability to recall everyday words, and memory loss. (webMD)

Brain fatigue and fog can be some of the more invisible, harder to recover from effects of having a brain injury.

I think it's kind of something I'm fine-tuning as I learn more and more about the body. I just became fascinated with the brain and stroke recovery. As most stroke survivors know, you must make your own path, everyone is different. There is no set way to recover from a brain injury.

I've learned through yoga and science that we have a reptilian part of our brain, located in our brainstem, or the oldest, most primal part of our brain. This is our default or factory setting. Our brain is hardwired to go to the negative thing first. This is not a "bad" thing. This is survival and probably the reason humans have yet to be extinct. Love envelops us and holds us, but survival is what we are born into, so to speak.

Our brain first sees everything around us as a threat. Everything. Safety is learned. Love itself can often be conditioned to be a threat.

It is only until we experience the world and start to examine what feels safe that we begin to evolve or grow out of this threat stage. This can happen at any time, and trauma brings a person right back into this survival mode, factory reset very quickly. Some might call these "triggers." No matter how much time passes, often one word, one smell, place, or time can bring the body right back into that visceral state of do or die.

If we graduate out of this primary thinking response, we raise our level of thinking into our higher consciousness or the neocortex. This is a higher-level thinking part of the brain that can cognitively process thoughts and sort through actual threats and perceived threats. The brain is processing and perceiving experiences constantly throughout our day and filtering them and sending messages throughout our body via our nervous system, through this huge network in the vagus nerve.

It is sending messages throughout our body all day, every second about how our body should behave in each moment. Responsible for attention, thought, perception, and memory, our neocortex is the biggest part of our brain. How should our body respond? Fight/flight or rest/digest?

Beyond this neocortex, we move into the pineal gland or third eye part of our brain that helps us see what is unseen. Only if the human desires to go beyond the abstract, physical thinking mind into this unseen realm does this pineal gland activate. You know how some people can see auras? Their eyes are untrained, so to speak. Their third eye is open.

For many of us, this gland remains shut through each lifetime. A stroke is an incident that scratches away all the muck that blocks this third eye and gives us an insight deeper than anyone could imagine. The pineal gland's primary job is to maintain the circadian rhythm of the body and produce melatonin. The National Institutes of Health define the circadian rhythm as "the 24-hour internal clock in our brain that regulates cycles of alertness and sleepiness by responding to light changes in our environment." I say this is our body's natural regulatory software. It is a neuroendocrine organ, part of our brain said to have energetic, mystical associations with the spirit world.

Every stroke survivor I have met has had this sixth sense of the pineal activation, so to speak. Some examples would be being more sensitive to light and needing more sleep regulation. This crack of an opening, whether they know it or not, "the crack is where the light enters," as the poet Rumi says. "A stroke switches you from unconscious to conscious living," stroke yoga student Swathi Roa describes.

This perception component combined with our human body's complex nervous system shifting in and out of rest/digest and fight/flight all day can greatly affect our actions, personalities, and behaviors without even consciously being aware of it. Lots of people are completely unaware of these shifts within their own body. The scary part of it is your unconscious mind guides pretty much all of your life, but most people aren't even aware they have an unconscious mind,

It is so subtle that it often goes unnoticed.

Evolution has everything to do with it. Humans are living, breathing creatures, not solid matter. We are ALIVE. We are made to move through life, change, and adapt. Our environment greatly impacts this level of change or sometimes a lack thereof. Every generation is slightly different from the last.

Change is what we are designed to do to at our innate state of beingness as humans. We are alive, pulsating, vibrating, oscillating beings.

I'm going to science geek out a few times here.

The human nervous system is made up of two major parts, **the central and peripheral**.

The central nervous system is the brain, spinal cord, and nerves. The peripheral nervous system sends messages outside the brain and spinal cord, communicating with the rest of your body. It houses our **autonomic and somatic movements.**

Our autonomic system controls involuntary functions: heartbeat and organ and gland function.

These things we don't have to consciously think to do, our body just does it. Somatic function includes voluntary movements and our senses.

These two categories are subdivided into more specific categories called the **parasympathetic** and **sympathetic** divisions of both the autonomic and somatic systems in the body.

The parasympathetic system is our rest and digest function, producing relaxation in our body, slowing our heart rate, lowering blood pressure, and increasing digestion. This system also controls salivation, tear production, digestion, urination, and defecation.

On the other hand, **our sympathetic system** is responsible for fight or flight, or fight, freeze, flight, our perceived danger response we talked about in the reptilian brain, preparing the body to be ready for a threat. It literally increases heart rate and slows digestion.

These two systems work in an ebb and flow all day long. Or they should at least.

I mention this because many common disorders are caused by overactive sympathetic systems—high blood pressure, irregular heart-beats, and more as stated in *The Key to Self-Healing* by Dr. Andrew Weil.

Well, high BP and AFIB or irregularities of heartbeats are common signs of stroke. We are connecting the dots.

According to the National Institutes of Health, stroke is a neurological disorder. Why are we not treating it as such? Nero physical therapy does not belong in a gym setting. This is counterproductive.

This basic knowledge of the human self is important when we do yoga and wonder why after a stroke the body seems to resist relaxation or almost prefer to be always in a hypervigilant state. Spasticity is a hypervigilant state of tension in the body, making it very hard to relax, not a muscular condition.

It is because the nervous system is overloaded and cannot move into a parasympathetic state; it gets stuck in sympathetic mode. It has nothing to do with weak or tight muscles as the medical community would have you believe. The solutions that Western medicine asserts are repetitive muscular exercises, surgery, and harsh pharmaceuticals. None of which can access the subtle network of nerves tucked away in the nervous system.

Harsh pharmaceutical drugs, unprocessed stress, noise, stimulants, and toxins can all put an added load on the nervous system. Trauma itself or an unexpected scary incident can be enough to throw the nervous system completely out of whack and in need of more consistent reminders to relax. It's all about balance for the sympathetic and parasympathetic systems. They work in tandem. Often, incidents in life affect the balance these two systems possess.

We remind the body to relax by accessing this subtle body and communicating with our body internally, in a subtle, quiet manner, usually by using the breath or soft touch, weighted holds, hugs, and things of that nature. Nervous system healing can be accessed through yoga, slow somatic movements, sound therapy, color therapy, heat or ice therapies, and actual nature!!! These are all subtle resources denied to those healing from a brain injury.

Not to talk too much more about the geeky science stuff I've accumulated in my brain from numerous yoga trainings and readings, but the brain is made up of three main parts. To recap: most ancient to most recently evolved, all branching into two main components of our nervous system, subcategorized into a lot of confusing departments.

You ever wondered why they don't start teaching this to young kids in school? Yeah, me too.

This is another topic of conversation for those interested in digging deeper into societal problems that keep the masses ignorant of their own spiritual nature.

- **Primal or reptilian brain:** What we are born into. Survival in the brain stem. Willpower is located in the middle part of our brain (basal ganglia and upper part of the spinal cord), our innate will for survival is here. Trauma can impact how often the brain uses this reset setting, particularly unhealed trauma.
- **Limbic brain:** Emotions, memory, motivation. Located in the hypothalamus, hippocampus, and amygdala.
- **Neocortex or cerebral cortex:** Sensory perception, conscious thought, language. As in higher-level thinking and reasoning. This is in a way a part of the limbic system in terms of locations; however, it is my understanding that as this part of the brain strengthens or grows, the reptilian brain shrinks. Eventually, possibly evolving away from the use of the primal area of the brain.

That is, of course, if trauma does not continue to significantly impact the brain. When love is withheld or absent and healing trauma is avoided, people can get stuck in this primal state, perceiving everyone and everything as a threat.

References: *The Brain That Changed Itself* by Norman Doidge MD; *Waking the Tiger* by Peter Levin, PhD and NDNR (naturopathic doctor news and review), or resources such as Sciencemag.org.

Back to love: Where it all begins and where it all ends. Love is a universal energy that transcends all those parts of the brain. Love is universal and where we came from and where we will return. We are literally bathing in it and it's oozing out of our pores.

If you, like many, grew up in a house where love or physical displays of love were scarce and conditional, you may often question this idea of love and struggle to love and accept yourself. Love is the baseline from which all existence is born. You do not need to do anything to achieve love or be loved. You are born loved, complete, and whole in every sense. All you need you have within.

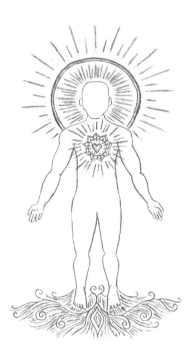

CHAPTER 2

TOXICITY

I have two children myself and I love my boys dearly, but you won't hear me say they are my world or my everything. I'm not giving them that much power over my life, nor am I pressuring them with my own expectations. This can be a form of toxic codependency and narcissistic control many parents exhibit, not addressed much in our society. We are all children of God, just visitors here. None of us really "belong" to anyone, neither in birth nor marriage. Children of stroke survivors are harshly forced to grow up very quickly and deal with things no child should have to face.

Young children can have a difficult time processing why the stroke parent is easily angered, tired more often, or forgets things frequently. The trauma this can cause in a young child is intense. Spouses often become caregivers and relationships often can be strained tremendously after returning home after a stroke. The guilt and shame of this for a brain injury survivor is so intense. When someone survives a brain injury, they should be celebrated, not pitied. More support is needed for young stroke survivors, especially those with young children.

Yet I believe my children, who were five years old and three months old at the time of my stroke, will be more empathic, kind, and considerate humans in this world because of my stroke. All children are born uniquely individual, yet collectively connected. It can be very hard to think about the impact your stroke has had on your kids. The guilt can be downright overwhelming.

Children can often assume the role of a caregiver at a very young age as well, and this can be a very hard thing to adjust to as a family unit.

Nothing happens that is not in divine ordinance; nothing happens to punish or reward us either. Stuff happens and it's just up to us to adapt to it.

"Wrong" just doesn't exist, because our life is in God's hands to begin with and our lifespan is not ours to decide—trusting God's plan, no matter what.

None of us are getting out alive.

Death is not the ending, but rather the beginning of a new cycle. The spirit never dies, yet it is just recycled into the earth or another life or whatever you believe.

My parents separated when I was six and my father made the choice to move out, leaving my mother, sister, and I to find a new way.

I understand why he had to make that choice as an adult, but as a young girl, I sat there with a blank expression as my parents explained he would be moving out. I felt hurt beyond belief to know my father would be living somewhere else, but I did not have the ability to express anything. I don't even think I cried.

My dad was never absent, he always came around and supported us financially. I know he loved us. Nevertheless, after getting the news my parents were splitting up, and sitting there dumbfounded, confused, silent, and in shock, our lives began to change rapidly. Things changed so quickly and continued to just change and change. Everyone seemed to hate each other more every day, and everyone just moved further away from each other into new worlds, not to mention they quickly became invested in dating and finding new partners. I had a hard time keeping up with it all, frankly. I wonder sometimes if my nervous system just didn't know how to cope.

The yelling, the crying, the tension always seemed to grow around my sister and me.

Not only did my dad move out, but I had to go spend time with him in this new apartment and "try to make the best of it."

The whole thing was weird. We spent time with him in his studio apartment. We played Nintendo and indoor basketball.

I knew my dad was trying his best to occupy us with fun things. It was fun. I could see how hard he was trying.

But it was at this time my goofy, silly self began to retreat inward. I began to occupy myself inside my own head. Little did I know, but I began my meditation practice when I was nine, using made-up scenarios to give my anxious mind a bit of peace as a way of self-soothing.

I came up with an alternate persona, Tiffany Houston. She was a famous "basketballer" or as I explained, a famous basketball star. She was rich and was very good at basketball.

In real life I played basketball a lot; it was my favorite sport.

Tiffany was created inside my head, and I even asked my family to call me that for some time.

The façade eventually grew tiresome, and my parents thought I was so cute and creative for concocting such a cute story. Tiffany served her purpose and was retired in the basketball hall of fame. She got a plaque and everything!

But as I grew, my ability to disassociate from my real life into an alternate universe grew and grew. My mind became a place I would often retreat to, and I introverted my personality completely as a pre-teen.

Tiffany no longer existed, but I became a teacher at nine and designed a whole classroom of students, homework, grades, parents, and the life a teacher might have complete with wardrobe, wallet, and apartment. As the world around me rapidly changed, my mind became a safe place to retreat, establishing lifelong patterns of being "all in my head."

Imagination play became my favorite pastime for years and years, well into my teenage years.

Imagination and creativity are gateways to the divine, but they can also be the root cause of developing overthinking patterns.

Little did I know, I was planting the seeds for the teaching degree I would eventually complete.

I became a teenager who rarely spoke. I retreated deeper into myself, feeling alone and misunderstood. I had few friends, and I grew angry and distant, and nobody really seemed to notice. I had always been a quiet, silly one, everyone said. I never needed much to be happy.

I knew how to laugh at myself. Even as a baby, my parents said I was just always content. But I grew deeper into myself as time went by and had so many emotions no one understood and often displayed emotions or opinions those around me found rude or offensive. When I did speak, someone was usually hurt or offended. My parents' own emotional outbursts were often perceived by me as being bothersome. As a child who felt emotions deeply, I felt all the tension around me, all the time. I noticed scowling faces and short, aggressive tones. Where was the love? Toxicity often is simply the absence of unconditional love. I had no coping mechanisms. "Gentle parenting" or child therapy was just not a thing in the 80s. A lot of parents lacked the tools to understand their children's emotional development.

I parted ways from a quiet child looking for validation to a teenager who did not care one bit, looking for validation in all the wrong ways. I went hard with fake IDs, stealing, drinking, and at nineteen becoming pregnant with my first child.

As I hear myself ramble, I am reminded none of this really matters. All families have trauma, no one is without suffering in this world. I only speak about this to show how my spirit began to hide inside my body and how I lost sight of myself at a young age, culminating with a stroke as the top of a shaken-up bottle popping off.

The number of stories I have heard from fellow stroke survivors about how they were going hard, working like crazy, up to their necks in something, then bam, stroke. It is not just my story.

We are unpacking these subtle themes.

Only after my stroke did I begin to unpack the "whys" into my own tendencies. Unpacking this trauma and acknowledging toxic behaviors or tendencies has become the biggest part of my healing and restoring movement in my paralyzed body. Often, trauma or toxicity get stuck in our body as trapped unprocessed emotion, although we may not remember or even think it matters. So many get stuck in the physical realm and ignore these unseen factors affecting the subtle body.

Stroke is literally referred to as the invisible disease. Yet so many invisible signs and symptoms are ignored.

It took my brain incident to shed light on some of these hardships that still live inside of me. My body began to physically tell a tale.

Our body remembers everything.

Many think the past is in the past so leave it there, but our body is a physical recollection of every experience we have ever lived through. I have learned through reading so many books on the brain that the body literally keeps the score, as MD and trauma expert Bessel van der Kolk describes in his book titled *The Body Keeps the Score*. You see, our body remembers everything we see, whether we want to or not; so my motto has become better out than in.

Love is not really an act at all, it is a frequency, it's less of a verb and more of a noun. It radiates from the inside out. I don't think many parents truly love themselves before having kids. So if parents are not attuned to this love, how can they properly give their children the love they crave? It's like how do I tune in to a specific radio station—I change to that channel. If I'm not on a channel, I may never know it exists or experience what that channel has to offer.

Love is a well, a frequency, a radio station, so to speak, felt deep within your soul, a connection to the God self or divinity within, a true acceptance for yourself.

"That my birthright is an infinite ocean of existence, knowledge, and bliss."

Reading spiritual texts such as *Pathways to Joy* by Master Vivekananda reminds us of this pure, perfect divinity within.

To give it or receive it, you need to feel the well within your own heart, something traumatized people have a hard time accessing. I know I sound weird, but I'm embracing it. I too have had difficulty accessing this heart center. In our modern culture, these ideas are often perceived as being selfish and full of yourself.

This could not be more false!!

I don't think these are things older generations are aware of. Loving and accepting yourself, taking care of your needs, and mental health days weren't a thing back in the day; it was go, go, go. I can respect that. But that is not the life of a brain injury survivor. Often, it takes a stroke to slow us down. And even after a stroke, it can be hard to embrace a slower, gentler pace, as therapies are often three to four times per week and rest is perceived as lazy.

Within my family unit and many others, many kids grow up alone or very misunderstood. We were told things like we don't talk about that, you weren't raised that way, or we don't do things like that, wear that, watch that, eat that. Control is often perceived and masquerading around as love.

Control can impact the psyche far more than anyone could imagine, always feeling less than, confined, and restricted.

When I became pregnant unexpectedly at nineteen, I had reached a point of no longer caring. I had been looking for love in all the wrong places, and becoming pregnant was the jolt into reality I needed. I decided to be a mother and change my life.

I often say my oldest son saved my life.

I decided to make my own path and do things the unconventional way. Completing my college degree with a toddler at home, I decided to make myself a priority as a young mother. I was again met with much criticism and called selfish for choosing to put my child in daycare.

I would have never had the courage to go to university as a single mom without the help of my father and stepmom. I worked my butt off to be the first in my family to receive a bachelor's degree. My degree was in elementary education with a minor in history, and I was off to tackle the Chicago public schools.

This writing is a huge piece of my own healing. I cannot suggest enough to you to self-reflect, get a journal, and write about the significant experiences that shaped you. Do not wait for a stroke or heart attack to begin to dive into the self. Stroke yoga is not just for stroke survivors. It is for anyone a little skeptical about beginning a yoga practice or anyone interested in awakening on this spiritual path.

Because of being the different one—the one that was called too sensitive, thinking about things most don't, spending too much time in my head—it was as a teen that I began to develop a complex that there must be something seriously wrong with me, and that continued into adulthood.

Still, to this day, often when I make a mistake, that "what the fuck is wrong with you, you stupid idiot" voice creeps in. Being met more frequently with loving awareness and a kind voice is a lifelong practice for me. Self-compassion is freaking hard and something that can feel strange and new, especially if chaos has been all you've ever known.

So many in the world have a difficult time dealing with death, whereas I was always just like well, it happens. My understanding often came off as insensitive to those around me, further creating a divide.

Death is the ultimate goal, right? Liberation of the soul, right? We literally begin the dying process from the moment we are born. We are all dying as we speak, "walking each other home," as Ram Dass so eloquently says.

Nobody is getting out alive, right? To fear death is really confusing to me, especially from religious people. This idea that once you have a cancer diagnosis, you are going to die is nuts to me.

None of us know whether we will live to see another day EVER, cancer diagnosis or not. I even hate the word cancer. All cancer is a cell that divides. Why do some cells rapidly and uncontrollably divide? Well, look around you. This modern lifestyle breeds poison that remains lodged in our cells, causing confusing internal communication.

Cancer has become a dirty word, when it's a natural process of the cells. It's not a disease; it's a process within the body.

Cutting it out immediately only aggravates the body further. Garbage air, garbage food, and negative thoughts that fuel these so-called "cancerous" cells lose their role and go crazy. They can also be corrected somewhat easily.

Yes, I believe that "cancer" is definitely 110% "curable," but "cure" is not the right word, because it's not really even a disease, it's a process. It's more like restoring health to the cells, not "cure." It's bringing the body back into homeostasis and finding balance. No one will ever find a cure for cancer because there is no cure. It is a restoration to homeostasis. Homeostasis: equilibrium, regulated internal conditions remaining stable and constant. (National Library of Medicine). It is easier for our bodies to be healthy than ill. We just have a habit of getting in our own way.

I'm not sure if our culture will ever change here in America. But overseas, treatment is very different. Pharmaceutical companies have made cancer a billion-dollar industry, but maybe change is coming.

To cure anything is ignorant terminology; you must get the body back to balance. Yoga, music/sound therapy, dietary changes, meditation, and gentle things can do this. Yes, music or sound is the medicine of the future, to quote Albert Einstein. Big pharma is not something I trust, and I speak of the cancer industry because it goes hand in hand with the stroke industry.

Stroke recovery consists ONLY of surgery, PT, medicine, and robotics—all kinds of technology—when what the brain needs is peace to heal itself. Peace and relaxation are healing. Why can't there be a balance between modern and ancient healing practices?

This toxic surgical, medicinal culture is what I hope to change by completing this writing or at least open up a conversation.

Accessibility to healing tools that actually work is key for anyone dealing with disease or changes in the body. We should not only have access to Botox as stroke survivors. We should not get told to go home and figure it out.

Tell me why harsh pharmaceuticals are my only option?

Tell me why I'm denied treatment or often turned away from PT centers and yoga studios and shunned from society in general, when there are modalities such as Thai massage, sound baths, cranial sacral, rolfing, breathwork, yoga, and meditation that can be used cost-effectively and somewhat easily and noninvasively. Where are my choices and support for recovering from this massive event? And why if stroke is the leading cause of long-term disability, why aren't we looking at the rehab model?

Stroke survivors deserve less invasive options at the least. You don't have to love all the natural healing things I do, but options should be available. You should not be banished to the shadows to live a disabled life forever.

Brain cells cannot remain dead in a living, breathing body. There is, after any number of years, hope to be found within the human body. After fifteen years my hand is becoming more functional. I work with stroke survivors of all ages and races that begin to see results in the first yoga session.

While my expert stroke doctor told me I should be happy to be alive, without regular Botox, surgery, or baclofen, I had no chance of relaxing my spastic hand. Go figure.

Regardless, the notion that poison, i.e., pharmaceuticals or surgery, will restore balance in the body is a little nuts to me, but everybody is different. I remind myself of this daily.

Yes, I've had elective surgery before, so I do believe in modern medicine to a point. I am appreciative of many of my medical professionals. But medicine cannot "heal" a damn thing. It only masks one symptom and causes 12 million more issues, clogging up the bodily system with toxins. You're going to use a neurotoxin such as botulinum toxin-A to help restore the body after a stroke? Why? It's so counter-productive. It bloats the body and creates further fogginess in the brain. Two things that make recovery harder for stroke survivors.

I think all people are entitled to do whatever they want. But why the medical professionals decided a neurotoxin was a great idea for re-ducing spasticity after an injury to the brain seriously boggles my mind. I think it is medical negligence.

The beauty of life is we all get to make our own choices. I would never judge someone's choices to use medicine or surgery if that's what they feel is best, but I cannot stand by and be silent knowing this whole other world of subtle resources is out there and everyone is minimizing or straight ignoring it!!

Why can't I just go along with life and keep my big mouth shut? Why has my health forced me to dig deeper? Why can't I just live a more simple-minded existence and not question life so deeply?

Often when we want something so much, we start to control the outcome and limit ourselves tremendously from our full potential. But in the most poetic way, once we release it into the universe it finds its way to us. Holding on and letting go might be this dance of life we call yoga.

I'm reminded of **Sthira and Sukha. Steadiness and Ease.** How long do we hold and when do we let go?

How do we maintain a natural/steady Rhythm of life.

As an Abraham Hicks fan, I strongly practice the laws of attraction and wish someone would have told me about these universal principles of the universe a lot earlier. My lifestyle may never gain full acceptance.

Yoga is my health care, nature is my medicine, love is my religion, thoughts are things, and pleasing thoughts are all I have room to entertain. Poisons in my body are limited.

In a modern society, this can be nearly impossible to maintain. You are harshly judged as being weird, crazy, careless even.

Older generations were taught to respect their elders no matter what. As humans evolve, my generation and my children are taught more to use their own minds, question things, recognize their own limited base of perspective, and truly honor another human's experience, learn how to say no and where and how to draw a boundary.

Many households were and are lacking love. It has only been since the millennium that people have turned more to love and acceptance as a natural state of being and not a conditional force put upon us. There's still a lot of work to do.

Having the courage to move out of Chicago after my stroke as a grown woman was the single best thing I have ever done in my life. I literally never felt like that was my home. It's odd to be born into a life that feels so foreign and cold.

I think we need to be moving toward healing and get away from these "toxic" traits. Toxic meaning poisonous, unpleasant, abusive even. Toxic is a word our current culture loves to throw around.

This definition is true in a way, but this definition does not satisfy me; it is much deeper.

When I refer to someone as toxic, it means they are in need of healing. Said "toxic" person has not taken the time to heal from traumas they came into this life with, or traumas inflicted early on in life, so they have developed certain behavior patterns that lack clarity in the mind. They have a deep disconnection to their true self. Sometimes trauma can be suppressed and ignored for years, making it almost impossible to heal because you almost don't even consciously know it's there. However, negative behaviors develop out of this unhealed trauma, and to describe the behaviors, we use the word toxic. A toxic person can have wonderful traits, as well as toxic patterns and therefore, toxicity can become even more confusing.

Unresolved trauma creates a kind of disconnect in which everything (the mind and body) operates from a natural self-protection mode, overactive ego, excessive pride, or narcissism. It's that reptilian brain taking over. Everything becomes about your survival and further isolation occurs, replaying lies in your head (telling you people don't actually like you or are out to get you). Trust me, I know.

I think we ALL can exhibit narcissistic behavior at times.

Toxic traits such as:

- Overly emotional responses
- Lack of emotional self-regulation
- Gaslighting/distorting reality
- Arguing and instigating, yet walking away claiming innocence
- Excessive pride

- Demand for something
- Lack of involvement or over-involvement
- Lack of healthy connection
- Absence of healthy sharing/no judgment-free zones
- Expectations
- Codependency
- Judgment
- Assumptions
- Forced tradition in the name of family
- Forced apologies
- Power plays with other people/taking sides/excessively demanding loyalty
- Diminishing feelings/suggesting things could always be worse
- Extreme emotional attachment to certain words
- Comparisons, like this is worse than, or this is better
- Responsibility for others' feelings
- Interrupting/not listening
- Ruminating on certain words or phrases
- Imposing guilt
- Gossip
- Playing siblings against one another
- Shaming: What's wrong with you?/How could you?/That's not how you were raised
- Excessive EXCUSED negativity: "Oh, that's just how they are," "Don't take it so seriously," OR "You're being too sensitive."

- THE IDEA THAT YOU CAN MAKE SOMEONE ELSE HAPPY (**happiness is an inside job**)
- People-pleasing
- Smothering
- Overbearing
- Helicopter parenting
- Attention-seeking
- Explosive outbursts
- Uncontrolled anger/rage
- What-if scenarios
- Jumping to conclusions
- Racism/sexism
- Overly firm boundaries (Yes, boundaries are great, but not being flexible can be a very toxic trait.)

I'm sure we could all add a few. The list literally grows longer every day humans walk this planet. What might have been ACCEPTED or unnoticed behaviors at one point in time have evolved into a deeper examination of things, and that is a really positive thing for this earth and the human race in general. This is the evolving nature of life: Things change. Growth will change this world.

Add your own possessed or observed toxic traits:

....

....

....

Most humans exhibit these behaviors. They are learned behaviors and, therefore, can be unlearned. Seventy-five percent of the population is traumatized and 1 in 3 will exhibit toxic traits in a lifetime. I, myself, am not excluded.

This unhealed trauma causes many undesirable traits and can breed deeper issues such as excessive pride, EGO, narcissism, bipolar disorder, depression, or various addictive behaviors. Not because a person is "bad," but because suffering is going on in the body and there is turmoil. Lots of times it can create physical reactions within the body or chronic pain. All of these things can disturb the breath, and once the connection to the breath is disturbed, the connection to spirit is compromised.

Dr. Weil says breath is the *"movement of spirit"* within the body. Working with the breath seems to *"bring about spiritual awareness,"* he says.

He goes on to explain that "the breath is the only function in the body that can happen consciously or unconsciously." "It can be a voluntary or involuntary function." This is significant at the very least.

Dr. Weil confirms "working with the breath is good for everyone." I say for a stroke survivor, it should be mandatory right from the start.

"It is free. It requires no equipment and is literally right under your nose," Weil says.

When someone is exhibiting toxic traits disconnected from their spirit self, the person should be treated as if they have severe PTSD. Any exhibitable "poor" behavior can be understood from that perspective, not from a scolding perspective.

But as trauma often is ignored or untreated for years, even decades, toxic traits develop deeper and deeper, and it can make connecting with people very hard, nearly impossible sometimes. Not to mention that the discovery of epigenetics has taught us that trauma passes up to seven generations in our DNA, and certain genes can turn on and off in one's life. There was a man I watched an interview with who had his pointer finger cut off at ten years old, and twenty years later his daughter was born with a shortened pointer finger matching his. Epigenetics is powerful and explains why it is so important for parents to address their trauma before having kids because it will live inside their children.

One of my favorite Buddha quotes is, "If you like a flower, you pick it, if you love a flower, you water it and watch it grow." My hope is for humans to stop trying to pick each other apart and just love and watch each other bloom.

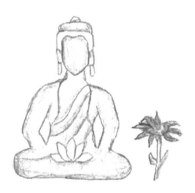

CHAPTER 3

SPIRITUALITY

You see, I don't believe "good" or "bad" really exist how they are perceived. I can be hurt or angry for the various ways I was treated as a child, but I don't think of anyone or anything as "bad."

I believe in the goodness inside each and every one of us. No, I don't think that makes me naive in any way. I believe humans are good-hearted by nature, and yet we live in a society that will do everything to get you to believe otherwise. Spirituality doesn't mean one thing or another, it is just embracing all that you are, living an authentic life, not bound by the structure of societal norms in some way.

Spirituality is just an unbound version of religion.

Each religion is not that different at all. They only complement each other, like different sides of the same mountain, as author Emmet Fox writes in his *Faces of God* booklet.

Every religion has a story, an acted-out version of this energy in physical form. How else could they explain it to the masses?

Jews had Moses.

Christians had Jesus.

Islam had Muhammad.

Buddhism had Buddha.

Taoism had the Tao.

Even satanic religions have something. Satanism worships the planet Saturn (the lowest vibrating planet), or if you believe in Satan as the fallen angel.

And Hinduism, the oldest organized religion, has many, many faces of God.

I admire all perspectives to a certain degree.

Religion is an unnecessary ideology, a construct. Personally, I'd rather go straight to the source. I can't help but wonder if the control religion has imposed has done more damage than good.

But none of this religious separation matters. **Everything is everything**.

Judgment is slowly dying as more generations detach from the physical focus of past generations and simply allow love to grow. In general, younger generations don't try to limit or categorize things as much as older generations.

I accept all of the world religions as valuable and have read many religious texts. None of them are **Truth** to me, for the only truth I believe in is that there is **one God, the divine, the universe, source, or whatever name you identify with**.

Not a "he" or a "she" or "it," just God—the one and only almighty one, not definable by a label or pronoun. God is everything and everywhere. God is not a thing, man, or woman. God is omniscient, a limitless energy source not limited or bound by any structure, and present with us wherever we go in our own hearts. God is not possibly a human, nor a judgmental figure in the sky. God is in me and you and the tree and the bee. It is so strange to think of God as a human.

God is good, and humans are reflections of God.

This means humans innately are good. The good will always outweigh the bad.

God is not a reflection of humans. Humans are a reflection of God, though.

This concept is very hard for the human mind to understand. We have been so conditioned to see the separation of God and man and have been taught that there is something wrong with us from birth. We have all been convinced we are sinful and flawed, and negativity does come "easier" into our brain because of the reptilian factor, but the thing about it is we are not "doomed" to live a life stuck there. There is so much light, good, and hope. You must move out of using that other part of your brain, redirect, and learn a new pattern. The science of this stuff is fascinating.

It's funny to me that people think of spirituality as woo-woo funny stuff when it's just science.

It's not whether we are **good** or **bad** as humans that is in question.

Good, bad, happy, sad. These are feelings in the body.

And a feeling is fleeting, it is a moment within oneself, and the cause has nothing to do with those around you.

You are worthy by birthright. Nothing outside of yourself can define you. No one can make you feel any sort of way. Our internal world sets the tone for our outer world, not the other way around.

As Rumi, the Islamic poet, so elegantly put it:

"Outside the field of right doing and wrongdoing there is a field. I will meet you there."

As Deepak Chopra says, "An emotion is simply a thought that creates a bodily sensation." And as Abraham Hicks says, "A belief is just a thought you keep thinking."

Thoughts strong enough to create a bodily sensation are not to be taken lightly. Feelings should never be denied or talked out of.

Deny them for what? Feelings are fleeting but at the same time are the way our soul navigates this life. Feelings are cues or signals.

In my belief, my parents were never "bad" parents, nor was I a "bad" daughter. Nor I am "right" and they are "wrong." I never really consider myself right about anything. Right creates a blockage to learning further. None of that exists by the confines we are accustomed to.

It is a different plane of relativity. It's not vertical. We have lived in a severely limited one-dimensional universe.

How do we know what is real? Blue pill or red pill? (A *Matrix* reference.) It is a horizontal plane, not vertical, the full expansion of the universe within us is truly a beautiful thing.

Yes, of course, there is a certain moral code, a successful way humans can live together on this earth in peace. Not the Ten Commandments or the threat of eternal damnation to get people to behave, but practices that, I like to say, make living on earth together a bit more bearable. Like the eight limbs of yoga (referenced in the yoga sutras and from my 200-hour teacher training and numerous books in print). One being *The Seven Spiritual Laws of Yoga* by Deepak Chopra:

1. **Pratyahara**: disconnection of outer senses, inner attention.
2. **Dharana**: concentration of mind, active focusing on one point, steadiness of mind (can be a form of meditation).
3. **Dhyana**: fully immersed in mental activity, there is no focused attention, being in the flow state, so to speak (another form of meditation).
4. **Asana**: physical posture.
5. **Yamas**: external practices to observe as we interact with the world.
    *   Ahimsa: Nonviolence
    *   Asteya: Nonstealing
    *   Satya: Truth
    *   Brahmacharya: Moderation
    *   Aparigraha: Simplicity
6. **Niyamas**: internal practices to observe.
    *   Saucha: Purity or clarity
    *   Santosha: Contentment
    *   Tapas: Discipline
    *   Svadhyaya: Self-study
    *   Ishvara Pranidhana: Surrender to divine
7. **Pranayama**: breath expansion.
8. **Samadhi**: full absorption to the divine.

These limbs are not in order, do not need to be done in any order, although Samadhi is the final absorption process—self-actualizing or self-realizing and fully connecting to the divinity within.

Letting go of all else.

Freedom is the ultimate goal of Yoga.

Of course, there must be a broad outline in which we monitor ourselves on this human experience: Sanskrit rules of life:

You will receive a body.
You will learn lessons.
There are no mistakes, only lessons.
A lesson will be repeated until it is learned.
Learning lessons does not end.
What you make of your life is up to you.
Others are simply mirrors of you.
The answers lie within.

My views are broad and maybe a bit weird, but it's not nearly as limiting as a big chunk of the population looks at it. It's more like general self-reflective guidelines based on the principle of innate human *goodness*, not rules or commandments.

People are NOT assholes, and the world doesn't suck. Life is pretty much your thoughts and attitudes manifesting into your own reality. However, due to trauma, a human can be taken away from this true innate goodness and exhibit asshole-like behavior, for sure!

It can be easy to get away from this true nature.

I don't believe in heaven or hell as locations, up and down, or being a good person to get to heaven. Living in fear of the threat of hell for doing bad things was something that absolutely never scared me, although I could see I was being pushed or literally forced down that road with my family. Not wanting to baptize my kids or force religion on them, I resisted the best I could, despite the judgment I received.

The devil does not exist outside of your own heart and mind either. He is not a "he" or a big bad anything, just as God is neither He nor She. It is not a vertical plane; Heaven up, Hell down. But the devil is darkness within your own heart-mind, citta-vritti, the second yoga sutra, according to Patanjali. The *Bhagavad Gita* tells us the mind creates bondage for humans. While yoga is a practice that frees that bondage.

Sutra I.2
Yogas citta vritti nirodhah.
The restraint of the modifications of the mind-stuff is yoga.

These *citta-vritti* or thought fluctuations (mind-stuff) often convince you of horrible, awful truths and make you forget the pure goodness inside of you. They'd have you believe you are unworthy or flawed, sinful, or "bad" upon birth. If you only knew the power thoughts and spoken words hold, you'd certainly get control of your mind and mouth ASAP. The mind is the second largest energetic source in the body, the heart field being the strongest; the mind is the more delicate, more easily influenced source of energy within.

In her book *Sacred Contracts*, author Caroline Myss says, "If people knew the true power of their own thoughts, they would never leave the house."

I say that as something I have learned, and I wish fewer people would force their own worries or words onto others in different situations. Often, young minds are filled with all kinds of things that are not reflective of the true nature of the human. The words often replayed in our minds are not even our own. From the time we are born, our minds are programmed by what we are told and exposed to, creating our thoughts and therefore creating our reality.

Heaven and Hell are *spiritual planes* we can create or free ourselves from in this life, and it can continue through multiple lives over. Lessons not learned here are repeated. I think anger is a sacred energy and deserves hearing it out or sitting with it.

Another toxic mantra is, "Why are you so angry?" Calm down.

What angers you in this world?

....
....
....
....
....
....
....
....

CHAPTER 4

ENERGY

I am finally learning to let go and move through things, to move stuck emotions through my body through the practice of yoga. It's freeing my arm up and relieving my anxiety and depression, plus improving my health, and increasing my energy levels.

Energy = Emotions

Stuck energy locked up in the body creates spasticity. Heavy emotions get stuck in the body, actually weighing the body down or making the body feel overly heavy. The reason is unique to each person. I say the breath is obstructed and there's no life force in the body; therefore, it assumes a heavy quality.

It could be an emotion, a heavy visitor that never left. It could be a breath blockage, nerve blockage, or spinal misalignment blocking flow of breath. The source of spasticity lives in the spine, not in muscular belly. This is a trend I have seen and needs further investigation. I would love to see our neuroscientists and experts study this further.

I believe in something called vitamin C flushes—a few times a year or so, flushing the body with a few hundred or thousand milli-grams—or daily rushes to jolt the body with electricity. I also think fasting could solve a lot of conditions within the body. When I do a vitamin C flush I basically take a ton of vitamin C to reach my max amount, and it creates a natural colonic. You use that amount every few hours for the rest of the day. It cleanses toxins from the belly and colon and refreshes the energetic function and flow of the body.

This has been known to "cure" cancer in some circles as well as fasting.

EVERYTHING IS ENERGY. It is all that matters. Vitamin C is like the juice for our body's battery, so to speak.

We don't naturally synthesize vitamin C. It is one of the few ne-cessities humans don't produce within their own body. Often, because of the GMO quality, our American food creates heaviness and confu-sion in the body. Fasting gives cells time to reboot.

No, I am not in a cult or occult. I am not a Buddhist, Scientolo-gist, Hindu, Muslim, Christian, witch, psychic, Pagan, heathen, lacking moral character, or a bad person, selfish, one-sided, racist, or uncaring. I refuse to be defined by any labels.

I left Chicago to find freedom and breathe deeper, to explore a different way of living, a softer, more conscious life.

Some wounds I didn't even know existed until I started unpacking. My breath is still deepening and it seemed like things just kept rising up and probably still will as this process continues. I had no clue it would take this long to unpack things, nor do I know why. Healing, just like experiencing a stroke, is a lifelong thing. You don't finish healing and then say you're done, you completed your healing, or you mastered yoga and now you can stop.

But as a part of my healing, I will never, ever apologize or regret:

- expressing myself,
- asserting myself,
- putting myself first,
- being different,
- having feelings,
- being sensitive, or
- getting upset.

And no human should!

It's important to remember: Ease is our natural state, the way we come into this world, completely perfectly flawed (perfection does not exist), at peace, whole, and complete in harmony— sometimes unfairly carrying past-life traumas. But it is the disruption of this natural state that creates places within the body that are disrupted states of ease, i.e., DIS-ease. Absence of ease.

Energetic disruption.

More Sanskrit words-

Sukha: "Su" meaning good "kha" meaning space. Good space, ease, gentle, mild, virtuous as yoga international describes.

Dukha: Meaning suffering, stress, dis-ease.

Our whole medical system and language are built on this ancient knowledge, wisdom, and Sanskrit language, but because of money and greed, health has turned into an industry. Suture, meaning to sew or stich, comes from the word Sutra in yoga. The health care industry completely confuses me. You are customers, not patients. There is no education of the brain or muscles after a stroke, no nervous system talk. Why?

Is it all really about the almighty dollar?

Health is in your hands only. So restoring natural balance while living in this modern society is really the challenge and the key to optimal health. Just imagine if we had more access to these wholistic modalities. No one would ever suffer from disease, and the billion-dollar pharmaceutical industry would plummet. Insurance companies would go under. Society itself would collapse.

We need more accessibility to nervous system, trauma–informed therapies.

But I'm afraid the powers that be will not allow such a thing.

When it comes to energy systems in the body, we know about the subtle system. Now we are talking about how energy moves through the body.

What kind of energy are we talking about specifically?

Vayus or winds or kinds of breath/life force energy that moves through the body.

There are five of these breaths that move along the spine:

1. **Prana**: chest, head, intake, inspiration. Base of throat to navel downward, clockwise motion. Upward counterclockwise from navel to throat

2. **Apana**: downward navel to pelvis, elimination energy

3. **Samana**: navel assimilation, discretion, inner absorption

4. **Udana**: throat, speech ascension, expression

5. **Vyana**: circulation, expansion, whole body

We have three major representations of these energies in our body: the seven main **chakras** (energy wheels), **Meridians or nadis** (more than 72,000 tiny little rivers of energy flow, known as nerves), and our **Aura** (the energy outside the physical bounds of our body).Our aura expands about an arms length outside each of our human bodies.

There are seven major chakras, although there are many more, and twelve major meridians on each side of the body. Three major nadis run up and down and side to side in the body.

The three major nadis run along the sides of the body, up and down, meeting at the spine with the chakras.

- **Ida** - left nostril, Yin energy, feminine, comfort.
- **Pingala** - right nostril, yang energy, masculine, tawny or fiery.
- **Shushumna** - center channel, joyful mind, good, virtuous, kundalini activation, energy up and down the spine.

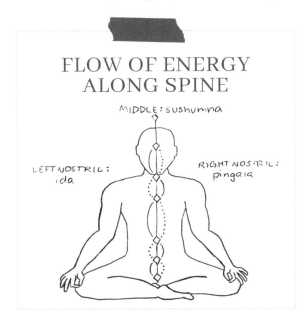

FLOW OF ENERGY ALONG SPINE

MIDDLE: sushumna

LEFT NOSTRIL: ida

RIGHT NOSTRIL: pingala

7 Chakras

- **Root (red) Lam** - base of spine
- **Sacral (orange) Vam** - reproductive organs
- **Solar plexus (yellow) Ram** - center of the body, behind aorta in the abdomen
- **Heart (green) Yam** - heart center
- **Throat (blue) Ham** - throat
- **Third eye (indigo) Ohm** - center of forehead
- **Crown (violet) Aum** - top of head

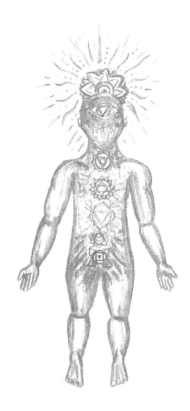

The meridians are split into Yin and Yang, being heart, pericardium, lung, spleen, liver, kidney, stomach, gallbladder, urinary tract, bladder, and triple burner (hollow space inside the trunk).

Now, in terms of yoga, there are two main ways to move or direct the flow of energy, mudras and bandhas.

Mudra: "gesture" or "attitude"

Attitudes of energy flow intended to link individual energy flow with universal.

These physical movements are intended to alter mood, attitude, and perception.

It may involve a combination of Asanas, pranayama, bandha, visualization, or in many cases be as simple as a gesture of the hands.

Mudras are a more advanced practice, accessing the subtle energetic body.

Linking the koshas (layer or sheath of the subtle body):

Anamaya kosha: physical body to Manomaya kosha: mental body to Pranamaya kosha: energy body.

In the *Asana, Pranayama, Mudra, Bandha* book by Swami Satyanada Saraswati, it is stated,

"Mudras manipulate prana the same way
that energy in the form of light or sound waves is
diverted by a mirror or cliff face."

There are <u>five groups of mudras</u>:

1. **Hasta**: hand mudras: for example, joining the thumb and index finger to engage the motor cortex at a very subtle level.
2. **Mana**: head mudras: utilizing the ears, nose, tongue, and lips to direct energy (gazing at eyebrows or gazing at nose).
3. **Kaya**: postural mudra: physical postures combined with breathing and concentration
4. **Bandha**: lock mudra—see below
5. **Adhara**: perineal mudra: lower sacral chakra pelvic floor: contraction and relaxation practice.

Bandha: "to hold," "tighten" or "lock"

In the *Asana, Pranayama, Mudra, Bandha* book by Swami Satyanada Saraswati, it is stated,

"Bandhas lock prana in particular areas and redirect the flow into the main energy channel of the subtle body."

Energy channels:

Ida: left/feminine energy/shakti energy/attributes dark to the Pingala: right/masculine energy/shiva energy/attributes light down the center of Sushumna: middle or central energy/balance/attributes generous and kind.

Four Main Bandhas:

1. **Jalandhara: throat lock:** bend the head forward so the chin presses to neck; breathe.

2. **Moola: perineum or root lock:** Contract the pelvic floor by bringing muscles up and inward. Contract tightly, relaxing the rest of the body and breathing.

3. **Uddiyana: abdominal or diaphragmatic:** Contract abdominal muscles inward and upward, hold and breathe.

4. **Maha: great lock (combining all 3).**

That's a lot of information, I know!

I need to add a disclaimer since I mentioned kundalini.

Kundalini is NOT sexual energy. Nor is tantra for that matter, but we will discuss tantra at a later time.

Kundalini is the energy running up and down the spine that is housed inside the base of the spine or pelvic bowl. It lies dormant until activated.

Any chakra can be sexualized. Any energy can be used sexually if you so choose.

The oversexualization of yoga is a very serious dilemma facing our modern society. Not to mention white-washing and often simply misrepresenting the tradition of yoga completely.

KUNDALINI (COILED SERPENT)
Life force energy along spine
We are all familiar with this symbol in the medical community
Coincidence or intentional?

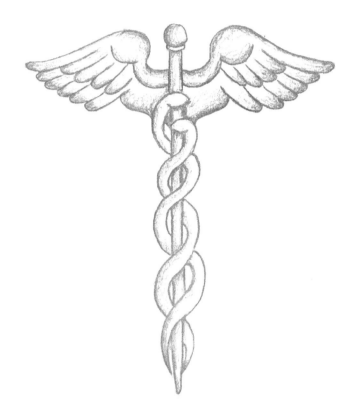

CHAPTER 5

SANTOSHA:
INNER CONTENTMENT

As I was saying, I was born with this kind of quiet inner niyama, or personal observance, contentment. Santosha, as we call it in yoga.

An inner knowing that all children are born with, I believe. We lose it as time passes though. It's a sort of forgetting that happens as a baby is born and grows up.

As content as I was as a young child, I grew into having this nagging frustration with life in general. I and many of us lose Santosha through experience.

I became a very nervous child and was often in physical pain, not always sure why. I grew irritable and unpleasant. Hugs were a rarity in my household. Anger was the predominant emotion. I often wonder what role that played in my physical health, as we know hugs are such a crucial part of hormone health.

It got worse after my stroke. As a child it was headaches, stomachaches, and sore throats.

What was the story with all the throat cultures in the '90s? The pushing of antibiotics was intense.

It was such a great way to disrupt the natural gut biome, as we have come to learn.

But since my stroke, I've gotten the headaches and stomachaches down for the time being, because my diet is strict and completely different. But now nerve pain, brain fog, and Nero fatigue have replaced childhood symptoms.

I dabble in vegetarianism, pescatarianism, veganism, and carnivorism. I don't really believe in strict restriction of things. I think supplements are the most important thing stroke survivors need right after the incident.

That is a good place to start, although everyone is different. As a young stroke survivor, I cannot emphasize feeding your brain the proper things enough.

Mushrooms in some form should be mandatory, in my opinion.

The study of psychedelics is another area we need to be exploring in terms of brain injury.

In addition to mushrooms,

- Zinc
- Vitamin C
- Selenium
- Magnesium
- TIME-RELEASED Iron (not for anemia but very effective for depression)
- Vitamin B6, B9
- Turmeric/curcumin
- NAC

- Vitamin D3
- Black seed oil
- Vegetable protein
- Collagen powder
- Algae DHA/ fish oil
- CBD

Cannabis in the form of green bud or flower, hemp, CBD oil, and RSO are all great safe alternatives to harsh pharmaceuticals. Just wait till we see how healing it really is. Did you know JFK smoked weed in the White House for back pain and other chronic medical conditions? That was probably why he was killed. THC itself can be linked to naturally thinning the blood and reducing repeated stroke in many cases.

Also, chia, flax, and hemp seeds. (When I'm on my period, I do seed cycling—a really neat way to balance women's hormones.) It helped me even out my cycle after my stroke. I don't think there is any diet that is best for all stroke survivors or all women or whatever, but supplements are often a rarely talked about process in the healing journey. Stroke survivors should have access to nutritionists, for sure!

Education about this brain/gut connection is key to stroke recovery. I'd go out on a limb to say spasticity is somehow related to the stomach lining and candida, as well as other overgrowths of bacteria within the stomach.

This is why I didn't continue with the yoga therapy program I had considered and enrolled in. I don't believe in generalizing when it comes to people or their health. It was not a program I wanted to be a part of. Yoga therapy is a field that compiles data on yoga and forms protocols in order to gain approval by insurance companies. Yet because yoga is so individualized, I wonder whether the field is helpful or limiting.

Right now, I believe migraine is the only condition covered by insurance for yoga therapy.

It is a growing area.

Because each human is so unique, I don't believe in categorizing. So, when I speak about what has helped me, please know it is just that.

What has helped ME.

Which is a very personal and narrow scope.

"The narrowness of my own experience," as Henry David Thoreau so eloquently describes in his book *Walden and Civil Disobedience*.

Mantras for inner contentment

The universe is conspiring for me and all I desire.
All that I need I have within.

STROKE SUPPLEMENT LIST

How are you supporting your body post-stroke?
List vitamins/supplements
Daily food log

CHAPTER SIX

AWARENESS

Now it's not the stomach or throat issues I'm trying to heal but the extreme nerve pain, brain fog, fatigue, and joint pain from residual wear and tear from my stroke and occasional stomach issues when my poor eating habits return. I was warned early on of the wear and tear, so to speak, that would be put on my body living with a stroke for the duration of my adult life.

Pain is something we can never avoid. I try to just take one day at a time and let myself rest when I need rest, without feeling bad for taking a day, laying low, or wearing PJs all day. Sleep guilt and supplement guilt can all be part of a stroke survivor's journey, with often those around us not understanding this somewhat "invisible" illness present some days and not others. It can almost seem as if it's a made-up occurrence.

But there is a difference between discomfort and pain. People can usually withstand far more discomfort than they realize before the mind backs out. We don't want to unnecessarily cause ourselves or others pain, but as my teenage son says, yoga is like purposely stressing out your muscles so they can naturally find relaxation.

The stress response is what we need for survival. Stress itself is a protection mechanism, not something we want to avoid.

When you step out of this physical realm and into the spiritual world, you start to build up an awareness within yourself that knows this spiritual being is divinely and universally connected at all times, without the limitations of the ego.

The words *I AM* are the two most powerful words. What follows them is a choice. In yoga, we call it a mantra. Claiming something. It is a meditation tool that can not only help focus or calm the fluctuations of the mind but is also a statement of ownership.

Mantra
Man-Tra
Mind tool
such as:

I am Peace,
I am able to calm myself with the ease of my breath.
I am Whole.
I am grounded.
I am worthy.

Mantra utilizes the two most powerful words in the human language.
I AM.
A kind of reprogramming of the mind.

A mantra is not a goal, it is a repetitive phrase you repeat in your mind, creating your own reality.

Goal-setting begins with thinking about where you are now and where you want to be in a few weeks. When you begin each yoga class, you begin with a promise or intention.

In Sanskrit, intention is the word **Sankalpa:** *a promise or vow we make to ourselves.* A quality you wish to carry with you through your practice.

Sankalpa is, what I would say, a promise you make when you set out, a promise to yourself. It remains the same day after day.

This promise is a quality you wish to cultivate or carry within your practice. This can be the same or different daily. Such as:

Compassion, Patience, Strength

An **intention** can be slightly more direct of a statement than a sankalpa or a quality we wish to possess, but the two are one in the same. Sankalpa is usually just shorter, a word, while an intention can be a longer setiment, however you feel inspired to inspire yourself. Intentions such as:

> *Every day in every way, I'm evolving.*
> *The universe supports my deepest desires.*
> *All is always working out for me.*
> *I am supported by a loving universal life force energy*
> *some like to call God.*

Kinda makes sense? Mantra, intention, and Sankalpa are all very alike, but different.

Yoga should always begin with an intention. A mantra and sankalpa can be cultivated as the practice takes shape.

The power of any of these can be applied to many other things in the form of "faking it till you make it," the act of demanding certain things based on the way you carry yourself, and your boundaries.

Within the construct of the mind when it is not in immediate danger, the ego is more or less the annoying little guy that keeps popping up to remind you it's there. The ego's job is to evaluate, label, and organize information coming in. But remember, ego is not bad or good. When it's a matter of life or death, the ego chooses life no matter what.

Different than most other species that would die simply from fright, the human ego protects at all costs. The ego will keep a human alive through some of the most horrid experiences. To reverse an over-active ego, recognition of trauma must be at the center of healing. Peter Levine, trauma expert, says in his book *Waking the Tiger* that the first step to healing trauma is spoken word.

Saying it out loud and accepting it for what it was. Kind of sounds familiar to AA, right? Yoga is all around us, whether we know it or not.

The kind of healing I'm talking about goes like this:

- Bringing awareness into the ego and speaking the trauma out loud, accepting it.
- Recognizing the ego and thanking the ego for all it has done to keep you alive up until this point. Do not apologize or allow a sense of shame for acts the ego may have committed.
- Make friends with the ego.

- The ego then will "go away" or be deflated as some say, and instead of leading ego-driven lives, you can live heart-centered lives. That connection I talked about that was lost is restored, and joy replaces all fear. State of ease is restored, and disease and pain eventually fall as the ego deflates, so to speak. Trauma heals.

Write a goal-setting statement of ownership of yoga practice, taking the goals from the beginning. The "My yoga will" statements:

Examples:

My yoga will help me evolve.

My yoga will bring me balance.

My yoga will help me find peace.

What is your mantra:

....

....

....

....

....

Changing these statements into Mantra to recite daily.

Sankalpa can be Evolving, Balance, and Peace.

I am evolving.

I am balanced.

I am peace.

Rachel Jarmusz

....

....

....

....

....

CHAPTER SEVEN

BREATH

I was a kid that yawned a lot. Why was I yawning all the time, what was wrong with me? It came off as very rude to others at the time.

I don't think I ever breathed right. My bottom rib cage is collapsed into my diaphragm because of my spinal issues, poor posture, and god knows what else. So deep breaths always took too much work. I fell into the bad habit of upper-chest breathing (which is anxiety breeding). This is a sign of the vagus nerve shutting down. Yawning is an attempt to re-spark that nerve after it has shut down and retreated into the body.

Feeling unsafe and scared so long in my own body and in the space around me, I developed patterns of reverse breathing, which also limits your oxygen intake. *The Science of Breath* or *The Oxygen Advantage* are two great references on the topic of breath.

We don't actually use oxygen as in we breathe in oxygen. Bigger breaths does not mean more oxygen to our muscles. Our cells are saturated with oxygen, often getting too much oxygen, creating a buildup of these free radicals floating around our system, cells with no job. Is this the cause of cancerous buildup, possibly?

We breathe in oxygen, which forces our cells to release CO_2 A slow, steady breath is ideal, regulating our blood PH levels, keeping the body in this easeful stable zone.

"The primary stimulus to breathe is to release excess carbon dioxide from the body," Patrick McKeon says in *The Oxygen Advantage*.

He further says, "We need the blood to release oxygen, not hold on to it . . . CO_2 is the doorway which lets oxygen reach your muscles."

I still don't always get enough oxygen in when I breathe, or so I thought. I need constant reminding.

Come to find out over breathing, mouth breathing, or generally taking in too much oxygen is more of the issue I found. After completing his book, I realized less oxygen intake is actually better for the body. Breath retention is a valuable practice, as in using a bandha, a lock, or a kumbhaka.

There are eight types of breath retention or Kumbhaka.

Whether you're holding on the inhale or exhale or in between, these practices are a more complex or advanced yoga tradition.

When the body is traumatized, the breath becomes shallower and more stuck in the upper chakras:

the head, the throat, or the chest, not making it down to the lower half to fully nourish the body.

Does your belly move in when inhaling or press out?

Are you a reverse breather?

Pranayama in yoga was commonly known to mean breath control, but after closer examination of the word, we find out it's less about control and more about expansion, making the breath slow and steady, but also deep and full.

In *The Science of Breath*, Swami Rama defines four qualities of breath irregularities.

1. Shallowness
2. Jerking
3. Excessive noise
4. Extended pauses in between inhale and exhale

In *The Key to Self-Healing*, Dr. Andrew Weil categorizes the breath with the same qualities.

I am the quintessential reverse breather, belly sucks in on the inhale, out on the exhale. Plus, I have low heart rate, a slippery pulse, slow circulation, and my blood doesn't oxygenate properly. Probably all causes of my stroke my Western doctors failed to address.

I'm always cold, not iron deficient, just a traumatized reverse breather with poor circulation. The research I have done since my stroke includes a link between sleep apnea and breathing disorders such as CPD as common causes of stroke. CPD is a breathing disorder with no steady rhythm and interrupted patterns.

But I had to read about it on my own and share the research studies on my website, or it is easily searchable on the internet. I also studied the effects of THC as a blood thinner.

www. Myyogawill.com

Yawning is a cool way the vagus nerve resets and craves a large influx of oxygen. Slow inhales and deep, longer exhales reset the vagus nerve, as well as humming, ice therapy, and general relaxation.

Some might say the vagus nerve itself is our soul nerve. It is the largest nerve in the body.

Stroke survivors often yawn a lot during yoga class. This is not a cue of tiredness but rather a sign that the vagus nerve is communicating relaxation to the nervous system.

It's the actual separation from this Divine source or God that is the real challenge, which is the same as being disconnected from a steady rhythm of breath.

As Dr. Weil states in his book, "The breath is the animated, non-physical aspect of our being." What is the nonphysical aspect of our being? Our Spirit. Our spirit is what connects us all to each other and what connects us to the divine.

Not being flawed or sinful, innately bad, or impure, going to hell unless accepting Jesus . . . it may have been easier to just stay in "paradise," to stay directly connected as the story of Adam and Eve illustrates, or the Hindu story of Shiva and Shakti (that's one of my favorites). However, God wanted varied expressions and varied experiences outside of paradise. God created humans to literally live through us, and that was not meant to be limited to the Garden of Eden.

This "fall of man," I believe, is also misinterpreted in many ways that have been very harmful to our society. This is why I teach yoga, to help people, no matter what religion or background they come from, to connect with themselves deeply, internally through the breath. Yoga itself is not a religion. It is the antithesis of religion, a belief firmly rooted in self, excellently paired with any religious ideology or belief system already established. It's so beautiful!

CHAPTER EIGHT

CONTROL

Stroke survivors often feel out of control. Their life is no longer their own, and why did this happen? How is this fair?

Well, it's not fair. As a recent college graduate, to have the rug pulled out from under me in a matter of seconds was the most unfair thing life could ever do to me, but whoever said this life was fair?

Reminding ourselves what we have control of can be helpful to these notions of feeling out of control. I still, after fifteen years, drop into a victim mentality. *Why me* thoughts are hard to shake. Feeling worthless can be downright consuming.

Reminders . . .

What I can control:

My words

My actions

My ideas

My effort

My behavior

What I can't control:

EVERYTHING ELSE!

CIRCLE OF CONTROL

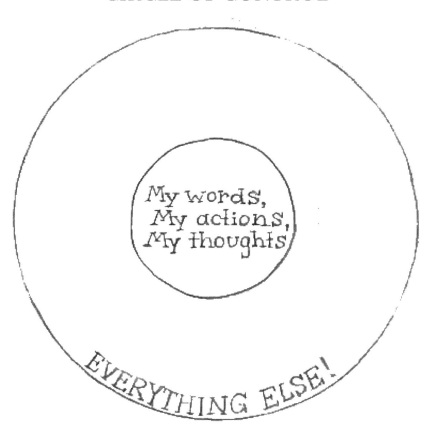

"I really don't care." Society sees not caring as such a bad thing whereas I think of it as freedom. Saying I don't care isn't a derogatory expression. I literally just don't care about so much. It is taken so literally and personally by many—but really, I care lots, maybe too much—but to me, I don't care means I don't have room for it and I have zero control over it so why fret. I literally cannot if it is out of my realm of control.

Often our own plate is full, and the world and those around us keep loading stuff on it. Plus, getting in the habit of letting what other people say about you influence you is one thing I really try not to do. Covid convinced our society we needed to care more about our neighbor than what we put in our bodies, and that's detrimental to society. We cannot take away civil liberties in the name of caring about our elderly neighbor.

Other people's opinions of you really don't exist, because their view of you is only a reflection of their own perception. What we see isn't reality, it is only a reflection of our own perception. It has nothing to do with you per se. Freedom truly comes when you no longer take anything personally and understand these concepts: Everything is everything, and everything and nothing matters all at once.

We are perfect, whole, complete, and also part of a bigger whole, all at once.

EVERYTHING happens for a reason. Once you absorb this truth, the victim quietly dies within and you are able to step into your own power, so to speak.

CHAPTER NINE

FEELINGS

I believe feelings are the only things we really have that are worth much in this world. However, they are fleeting, they can change very quickly, and although they offer insight into our soul's purpose, they can often be overemphasized and glorified as 100% fact, which is not healthy.

I am sad others make people think feelings don't matter, but they do, they matter. Feelings are like our little compass, guiding us to our true purpose. I honestly think God is involved, because I believe feelings lead us to purpose.

Go where you feel the most alive kind of a thing. Even if you think a feeling is inaccurate, you CANNOT EVER try to force it away/ deny it or tell someone to STOP feeling a feeling. Usually if you feel something unpleasant and bring attention to it, it moves through the body rather quickly. It's when we deny our feelings that we start to create internal issues. I think there is a link to emotional regulation and brain cancers.

Some people are invalidating someone's feelings or trying to convince them that what they feel is pretty horrible, or as many often say, "Just because you think you feel one way, doesn't make it so." How did society get so jumbled up when it comes to feelings? Possibly, generations of stuffing feelings down made us so out of touch with our own selves.

This manipulation of feelings has made things super-confusing to sort out as an adult. When you are always talked out of a feeling, you constantly doubt yourself. When those around you overspill it can be hard to even get in touch with your own feelings.

What do I even like? Who am I? I am only now discovering on my private island who I am as a woman and mother.

I have never been able to trust myself because I was always questioning my feelings and being talked in or out of something. Building a sense of self is so huge for a growing child and can help heal trauma. This would have been helpful to explore as a teenager, but I was denied that opportunity, not on purpose but kind of by default. My mother, too, had this dynamic with her parents. There was an overspill of emotions, making it confusing to sort out her own.

That is a really horrible thing to do, trying to manipulate someone's reality or perspective. (Again, this is gaslighting . . . feel what you feel and sit with it.)

If you can't trust yourself, then damn, who can you trust? I'm building up trust with myself, and it certainly takes time.

Yoga has helped me build my internal intuition, having little moments to check in with myself, just noticing and practicing nonjudgment, first toward myself then toward others. Yoga more than anything builds such confidence within, finding that deep, loving internal compassion for self.

My inner self grows stronger every day, little by little, so I know I'm doing something productive. The idea is we build up our own auras and get our own magnetic field really strong in order to manage this world more efficiently. The human spirit is the dopest thing on the planet. Our heart field energy is so strong, like a speeding Mack truck strength.

Nobody teaches us these things, though, so we are immediately at a disadvantage.

Being authentic means you honor your feelings, every feeling. Feelings tell us something, they give us insight, for sure; BUT AS A YOGI, YOU HAVE THE SELF-REALIZATION THAT YOU ARE NOT YOUR FEELINGS OR EMOTIONS OR THOUGHTS. YOU ARE THE SILENT WITNESS BEHIND ALL OF IT, I.E., THE SOUL that lives within the physical heart, which I do believe can have the power to tap into the universal God energy. Weird, I know, but true, our unchanging self.

I think it's how the pyramids were built and how Moses struck the Ten Commandments tablet in half. (We have limitless power and potential within that is directly from God, the divine source of energy.) I know a lot of my thoughts may appear weird or extreme to lots, but it feels amazing to explore my eccentric weird ways and build a like-minded community.

You see, the goal is for you to begin to separate from your feelings, *responding* to life, not *reacting*. I believe feelings connect us to our inner intuition and therefore build our internal connection to God. My theories are not scientifically proven . . . yet . . .but I am growing into organizing my thoughts. Being somewhat disconnected from the outer senses and internally dialed in so strong nothing can throw you off.

And mark my words, humans have not even tapped into this power. I might even suggest we have DE-Evolved through the years. As our society has become so modernized, we disconnected more and more from the internal self. But we will get back to it, I hope and pray.

For in this life there will be more hurt, of that I'm sure, and I can make no guarantees to anyone about anything. But focusing on the things I can control helps, as does doing the best I can in every moment, not expecting perfection but literally taking it one day at a time.

Every feeling actually links to a specific part of the body. If we studied somatic movement more carefully, we would find where every unprocessed emotion takes refuge in the body.

How do you feel right now? Practice articulating feelings into words.

....

....

....

....

....

....

....

....

....

....

....

Rachel Jarmusz

....
....
....
....
....
....
....
....
....
....
....
....
....
....
....
....
....
....
....
....
....
....
....
....
....

CHAPTER TEN

ANXIETY

Traveling, driving, opening windows, and being outdoors, particularly near beaches or mountains, relieves my anxiety because I feel like it's a breath of fresh air. I feel free, and it recharges me. I think anxiety manifests differently at different ages, and I'd like to explore that. Anxiety is such a broad term. It's hard to describe every kind, but anxiety is defined as a feeling of worry, unease. Dis-ease and un-ease are two very serious trends among humans.

Let's dive right into the doshas, or categories, that are believed to be present in the body and mind. The National Institutes of Health calls them brain patterns, associated with the three categories of regulatory behavior, according to Ayurveda.

My anxiety ramps me up, kind of like a very fast-moving mind. It's **a vata-pita** energy imbalance, fast-moving air and fire—the transformative/fast-moving kind of energy. Vata is really anxiety. It disrupts your natural state of ease but can manifest in so many forms.

My mother's anxiety is the exact opposite, more of **a vata-kapha,** a heavier more depressed state of anxiety often paralyzing oneself in the less talked about freeze response of the nervous system—maybe because of age or kind of trauma—I don't know. But anyone can find out their dosha by taking a quiz online. For example, Chopra Center has a good free one. It tells you a lot about yourself.

Basically, there are three main energy systems present within each human, according to Ayurveda, called doshas.

Ayurveda means science or knowledge of life. It is the ancient Hindu system of medicine, sometimes considered pseudoscience by critics of the ancient practice, that uses diet, herbal remedies, and yogic breathing to balance any overloads of stress causing havoc on the bodily system, causing dis-ease.

The doshas are based in the elements.

Vata-ether and air: cool, dry, light, irregular, rough, arthritis, anxiety, migraine, menstrual regulation.

Stroke is a vata imbalance. And most health issues are vata imbalance.

Pita-fire and water: hot, oily, sharp, soft, smooth, indigestion, heartburn, PMS.

Kapha-earth and water: cool, wet, heavy, dense, static, stable, depression, heavy sleeping, sick-a-lot kind of people.

We are made up of them and they are made up of the five elements: water, earth, fire, ether, and air. It's kind of cool because yoga reminds us that we are made of the same stuff as the earth. Pseudoscience?

Maybe.

There's a connection for sure; no one can convince me otherwise. That's why foods and herbs that grow in the earth heal our bodies so nicely. Also, nothing, absolutely nothing in nature is constant, it is always changing, so why would humankind be any different?

Ayurveda teaches us to adjust our bodies with the seasons and flow with life.

When it comes to creation, it's a story told through the Ayurvedic lense. The word Ayurveda translates to science or knowledge of life. It is the sister science of yoga, some might say, the science that backs yoga up. We have the creation story or idea behind creation being certain qualities or properties in the universe called the **GUNAS** coming together. These are less specific to humans and consider everything in the universe possessing these qualities. Not actual bodies.

Sattva: quality of pureness, positivity, truth, serenity, balance, truth, and virtue.

Rajas: passion or action, kinetic energy that results in activity, as One World Ayurvedic Institute in Indonesia describes.

Tamas: dull, sluggish, fear, avoidance, darkness, heaviness.

Anxiety can be still be anxiety and manifests in completely opposite ways. Based on these attributes and finding out the specific dosha of the person, so much can be discovered about yourself.

My anxiety makes me rush and feel like I'm always in a hurry.

So many types of anxiety in general have many similar qualities. General anxiety disorder broadly defined, has (which is what doctors have labeled me, with seasonal depression—to keep things really interesting) similarities that can include a heavy feeling, urgency, depressive states, and highs and lows. Any kind of anxiety having common themes:

- it creeps up on you,
- it tells you lies,
- it overwhelms you quickly,
- it rushes you needlessly.

Once you can identify these qualities, you can start to regain control of your thoughts.

Once you move into a brain injury and start examining some of the deeper brain conditions such as borderline personality disorder, ADHD, PTSD, severe anxiety attacks, or seizures, you dive into deeper realms of layers of thoughts and persistence of bullying oneself with one's own rapid thought flow.

Anxiety or depression can often convince you people don't like you or probably just hate you and think you are so ugly or dumb, or whatever your go-to negative description about yourself is.

That's why meditation is such a powerful and therapeutic tool, as someone who is healing my relationship with the way I speak to myself. Because of brain fog after a stroke, meditation should be a requirement for all stroke survivors, something taught in rehabilitation before being sent back into real life.

It really helps me feel safe within myself and questions some of this internal monologue. This feeling of safety was always something I searched high and low for. Always feeling unsafe with my family, building safety back into my body, maybe for the first time ever, is one way I'd describe yoga.

Yoga is you. How do I exist or "land" in my body?

Can I sit with myself?

Can I show up for myself?

Sit with yourself for five minutes and just breathe.

What comes up when you sit with yourself?

....

....

....

....

....

CHAPTER ELEVEN

STROKE

I had the discipline to finish college with a degree in elementary education after becoming a young mother. I had big plans, and on the way I decided to marry my then boyfriend and start a life together. Life was great!

We moved into a new city, had another child, and took in his two young toddlers. I wasn't able to find a healthy outlet for my stress, so slowly things got to be too much. All the pressure built up inside and came to a head on the day I had my stroke, shortly after giving birth to my second son. I think between my poor breath flow and imbalance of hormones post-partum, my brain had just had enough. The top popped off of a bottle that was shaken up for 25 years.

My stroke really saved my life, though. I had little self-awareness or spiritual backbone, passion, purpose, or meaning in life prior.

After two and a half weeks in the ICU, two weeks in neuro in the hospital, and thirty days of inpatient neuro rehab—where I had the challenge of relearning basic human tasks and reconnecting with a hemi-paralyzed body—I returned home to deal with the fallout, a failing marriage and young kids to tend to.

Recovery was difficult. I had a baby, a toddler, a husband in the military, and young stepchildren, not to mention career dreams that never came to be. Depression doesn't feel like a suitable word to describe the sadness I was left to manage. The anger, the rapid thoughts, anxiety, hemi-paralyzed body, brain fog, nero fatigue. Stroke survivors know this list is long and seems never-ending. Grief for the life I once knew still consumes me to this day.

Grief is literally a lifelong process.

I remember the day I returned home like it was yesterday. I wanted to be home so badly, and I wanted a shower in my own bathroom so bad. But I returned to what felt like stale, stagnant, heavy energy.

I looked around and saw memories of what felt like a different life. My family stepped up and offered to care for me full time, to help with both my children, and I made a bold decision to divorce my husband and make a new life for myself, recovering day by day.

I didn't feel I could get better in the same environment that made me sick.

If you really want to amp up your healing, changing your physical environment is one great way to do it. Often, we feel stuck mentally and we are stuck physically as well. Changing the physical environment can help the mental aspect catch up in many cases.

My stroke was completely unfair, caught me off guard, and turned my world upside down within minutes. But would I change it if I could? No.

Stepping out of your comfort zone is really what a stroke is all about. New neuro pathways, new ways of existing, new self, like shedding old skin and stepping into a new body. A different body albeit, but different can be exciting.

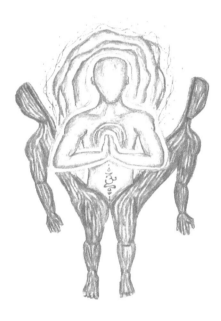

What beliefs are you stepping out of and reframing since your stroke?

....

....

....

....

....

CHAPTER TWELVE

YOGA

Rehab continued as I tried to piece together a life. My body was heavy, and I felt tired all the time. I did everything therapy and my doctors told me for five years, including surgery and Botox injections.

I was always met with, "We can't do much more for you, go home."

"Live your life, enjoy your kids, be happy you're alive," my doctor at a top-notch stroke rehab center told me one day as I was sitting in his exam room after wiping away tears from my eyes from the pain of the Botox shots I was told would help relax my spasticity. The shots hurt a lot and never did anything. So, I was questioning what I was doing, and I was met with the standard medical communities suggestions to stroke survivors: go home, live life. Since my own stroke, I have talked to well over fifty stroke survivors who have similar stories. Go home and do what, though, is my question?

Let's talk Yoga. How did it find me? No matter where I was, I was bored when I was in my PT sessions. One day in a session I was on a bathroom break, wandering the gym.

I stumbled into the medical gym connected to the hospital from my day rehab program, noticing a sign for a yoga class beginning soon. I stumbled up to the teacher, asking the teacher if I could do class with my hemi cane.

She was lovely. She welcomed me and set me up in the corner of the dark room. I had a huge hemi cane and leg brace.

I fumbled my way through the small class, barely able to keep up, the teacher encouraging me to just do what I could.

I experienced the purest state of relaxation. Upon leaving there, I was forever changed from that one-hour class.

I needed to know more about what I had just felt. What the heck was yoga? I continued to ask myself.

I decided to sell my home and move to Virginia in 2015, for a warmer, healthier climate, and start building a healthier lifestyle for myself and my sons.

We just did it. We began to make a life for ourselves in Virginia, absolutely loving living there. I began to do yoga with a very serious rigor two times a week.

I was walking better but I still used a brace on my leg; I still couldn't use my left arm at all, and I was dizzy, anxious, and depressed all the time.

Yoga really saved my life.

After a short time, I began to feel inside my body again. I began to develop a deep loving connection to myself. I have said before I wasn't just rebuilding from my stroke. I was rebuilding a life I never had. This time I was in charge. I was choosing thoughts, things, and activities that suited me, not anyone else. I began to put myself and my health first.

Conscious Living

I had to modify every yoga pose. I had to feel my body again or at least try. I had a beautiful, patient teacher who motivated me in a way no one else had ever done.

We worked hours a day sometimes on adapting a pose to my body. After a year or so of practice, I took a 200-hour teacher training to deepen my knowledge of the practice I was growing so deeply fond of. I never wanted to be a yoga teacher.

I didn't really want to be seen.

I completed my 200 hours in 2017 and by the divine grace of God started to be connected to other stroke survivors wanting to do yoga.

I have spent the last eight years doing and teaching yoga and taking more and more workshops to broaden my scope and fine-tune my craft.

I have decided to write about that journey and share stroke yoga with more stroke survivors, and it has been the most fulfilling thing I have ever done in my entire life.

I am so blessed to have had my stroke and feel grateful for the subtle changes it has made in my life.

PATANJALI IS CONSIDERED "THE FATHER OF MODERN YOGA." He may have been more of a consciousness than an actual man. Not because he invented yoga, but he was one of the eighteen classic Indian Sages and an intellectual conscious stream that took wisdom from the **VEDIC TEXTS** (HUMANS' EARLIEST LITERARY RECORD) and refined these ancient Vedic principles into text and direction—a more than 1,000-year-old text that gives us direct direction to yoga in 196 SUTRAS OR " THREADS."

Yoga can be referred to as many things, such as *the path to enlightenment or knowing the true self, realizing your true divine nature, or self-actualization. Yuj, yoke, union.*

How did yoga then reach America?

In 1893, Swami Vivekananda left India to come to Chicago.

The World Parliament of Religions, or the "World Fair," in Chicago welcomed the swami and his Eastern philosophy of union and oneness.

Vivekananda yoga is still in existence as a nonprofit organization out in California promoting healthy lifestyles using yoga.

There are many forms of yoga, but yoga itself is a path to self-realization, self-actualization, awakening, and beginning a journey within.

Here are some Broad styles of yoga:

- Jivamukti
- Bikram
- Anusara
- Bhakti
- Hatha
- Karma
- Tantra
- Viniyoga
- Chair

- Restorative
- Yin
- Raja

Modern society uses brewery yoga, goat yoga, core power yoga as ways to get this practice to the masses.

I believe any yoga in this world is better than none, although some practices make me scratch my head.

The eight-limbed approach or Ashtanga is the traditional approach to learning yoga in a more broken-down way.

The eight limbs to recap include:

1. **Pratyahara**
2. **Asana**
3. **Pranayama**
4. **Dhyana**
5. **Dharna**
6. **Samadhi**
7. **Yamas:** "right living," "reigning in," or "control"
   - **Ahimsa**: nonharming, nonviolence
   - **Satya**: truthfulness
   - **Asteya**: nonstealing
   - **Brahmacharya**: moderation
   - **Aparigraha**: nonpossessiveness
8. **Niyamas:** "positive duties" or "observances"
   - **Saucha**: purity
   - **Santosha**: contentment

- **Tapas**: austerity
- **Svadhyaya**: self-study
- **Isvara Pranidhana**: surrender to the Divine

Dhyana and Dharna are meditation. One with attention on and one with attention off a central theme.

So meditation is yoga and yoga is a sort of moving meditation itself.

Yoga is NOT an exercise!!

Meditation is this big umbrella word that has, along with mindfulness, become a sort of buzzword.

You know when you pause in your car and just stare a moment or look out a window for a couple minutes or seconds? Yeah, that's meditating.

No human is incapable of meditating. The industry itself has been built up under the illusion that you can be very good at meditating or not know how at all. Everyone knows how to meditate!

Humans are meditative by nature.

Listening to your favorite song as you drive to work, meditating. Gardening, meditating. Cooking, folding laundry.

Bring your attention to one thing and immerse yourself fully in it. Be alive.

Mindfulness is, simply put, paying attention on purpose.

CHAPTER THIRTEEN

STROKE YOGA

What is stroke yoga? What kind of yoga do you teach? are questions I get asked very frequently.

I say it is a combination of a few styles of yoga. You will see many different styles of yoga practiced in the world today, many different disciplines. Stroke yoga is a combination of:

- **Yin** yoga is a slower-paced, meditative, longer-held style of yoga within the Chinese tradition, designed to target deep tissue and increase flexibility.

- **Restorative yoga** enables deep relaxation, holding poses for longer periods of time without strain or pain, often using props, achieving ultimate physical, mental, and emotional relaxation.

- **Hatha yoga** means physical postures done and touches of vinyasa with elements of prop usage, as seen in Iyengar yoga.

- **Iyengar yoga is something I am not trained in specifically, but my own personal practice has become very Iyengar based. I strongly believe this community belongs with stroke survivors.**

The teachings of Iyengar are pure genius. I hope to continue to learn from his teachings.

My Yoga Will is the business I first began when sharing yoga. It was born out of my journey of using yoga as a tool for recovery after a stroke I had, in 2009, literally making this project more than ten years in the making.

With the focus on the latter half of my recovery, yoga wiggling its way into my consciousness about five years after my stroke, my hope is that all stroke survivors can access much sooner a system of yoga that works for their body.

I had one physical therapist in a hospital outpatient setting who introduced me, or I should say tried to introduce me, to "belly breathing," with no real context of practical use or explanation at all. Just lying flat on my back with her hovering over me, telling me to breathe into my belly. A concept I could not even begin to understand. I think PTs struggle bringing these concepts into their practice. This is a shame. Lots of Pts do yoga but struggle integrating it into their work.

She said I was a reverse breather. She never explained any more than that, and needless to say, I never saw her again. At the time, I never knew my journey would take me back to this idea of healing through breathing exercises. It's kind of ironic or poetic or something like full circle. I also had an occupational therapist teach me cat/cow poses, which happen to be one of the most fundamental yoga poses, with no mention of breath, but rather a lot of weight-bearing exercises with spinal extension and flexion. The attempts are there, but in my opinion fall short.

Again, I never realized these weight-bearing exercises were based on the whole system of poses, postures, and breathwork, its not just positions for the body. It was years after stumbling into my first yoga class when I realized yoga would embody both concepts that had already been introduced to me and tie them together in a practical, magical kind of way. I stumbled out of that first class and I was in love. But it took me years and a cross-country move to get me into a regular personal practice, preparing me for completing my teacher training and becoming a registered yoga instructor myself. It literally then occurred to me what a beautiful pairing. Stroke and yoga.

Having a disability and entering certain yoga communities can be overwhelming, and I understand why many don't. There are great teachers out there, but most yoga studios are just not equipped to handle this population without strange looks. If I wasn't thicker-skinned, I might have gotten hurt by certain comments and just left yoga behind. I think there are far too many benefits to walk away based on the ignorance of few.

I was told I would be better to go the adaptive route and utilize nonprofits, like accessible yoga organizations.

I choose to keep my yoga journey in the traditional route. Doing my 200-hour training in my local community and my 300-hour training at a Hatha yoga facility in Rishikesh, India. I think the goal should be more inclusive yoga across the board, not separate classes for those in need. The stroke population needs yoga more than anyone and yet gets ignored. I have chosen to be a visible reminder in the communities of this population.

Yoga is this complex system or practice that brings us into ourselves with love and compassion—healing from an injury that has disconnected us from ourselves or typically one-half of the body, breathing into the body because the disruption was all about blood flow and, therefore, oxygen loss. As I moved through my own yoga journey, I learned the fundamental breath techniques and postures and built myself up slowly, reconnecting to the part of my body that had felt so disconnected from the rest of my body for five-plus years. I had felt discouraged and frustrated in many ways, being so young when I had my stroke. After years of traditional Western therapy and medicinal treatments, I came to yoga as strictly a physical rehab for my body, knowing little about yoga and beginning in a gym setting like many do.

I found out along the way that yoga would not only be a way to help strengthen my body and increase flexibility but also ease the constant anxiety, low self-esteem, shame, and embarrassment I felt. This journey of recovery ultimately led me into deeper parts of my soul. Parts I may have never been in touch with to begin with.

You see, stroke survivors are some of the strongest, most determined group of people. The medical community has somewhat written us off as being disabled or "plateaued," putting limits on therapies and denying many forms of various therapies as measurable or valuable, not just yoga, but different energy healing and massage.

There are 7.2 million stroke survivors in the US, according to the American Stroke Association. That's a lot of freaking people!

Stroke is one of the leading causes of disability in the US, yet it is kind of ignored or dismissed by a lot of the medical community.

This has been my experience as a stroke survivor for fifteen-plus years now. I speak only of myself, with the hope that my journey can inspire others.

Slow, mindful movements combined with deep breathing techniques are used to reunite the body with the spirit. Many spiritual teachings suggest that when there is a severe trauma to the body, the spirit and the body separate. I truly believe this to be the case in my stroke. The breath gives us life. Andrew Weil writes about healing breath in his book *Breathing: The Master Key to Self-Healing*.

He speaks of the essence of breath as an expansion/contraction, a negative/positive, day/night, an oscillation of two poles.

He explains that it is what connects us.

Mimicking the stars and atoms, the expansion and contraction of the universe.

The breath is the animated, nonphysical aspect of our being, while the mind or the body is the concrete physical aspect of our being.

Our mind is so easily influenced and not always on our side.

Often, thoughts and words in our mind are not even our words or thoughts. Dr. Weil's work, for more than thirty years leading the way in integrative medicine, has used the breath as a sort of spiritual healing for the physical body. A bit pioneering, some people dismiss his odd tendencies, I know. It's not your traditional approach to healing, but it has been my experience that teaching yoga to stroke survivors is something worth digging deeper into. I have worked for years with various stroke survivors and have never had an experience with yoga not being helpful, yet it can feel like a sort of attack at first.

My healing is in my own hands? Huh?

Yoga is not for people looking to stay the same.

It can be an addition to traditional therapies and is most effective if used in a home practice. There is not a set of poses used for each session, although my program is designed around a specific sequence, which I believe is a good starting point for any stroke survivor.

Yoga is like building blocks of movement.

You don't really even need arms or legs to set the foundation, you just need a torso and breath.

Each yoga session is unique, just as unique as the stroke itself. Every stroke is unique; however, there are common "areas of vulnerability" after a stroke. This is what I call them, and they are unique to the person who experienced the stroke and dependent on the type of stroke they had.

Areas of vulnerability:

1. **Hip**
- Pelvis stabilization
- Hip flexor strengthening
- Hip openers
- How the hip and feet relate

2. **Knee**
- Hyperextension correction
- Hamstring strengthening
- Tendon release
- Joint-freeing series

3. **Ankle/foot/toes**
- Posterior kinetic chain activation
- Heel-toe walking
- Plantar flexion

- Toe relaxing/big toes pressing down
- Psoas activation

4. Shoulder

- Pectoral retraining
- Upper trapezius relaxation
- Scapula retraining
- Rear deltoid stretch and shoulder shrug
- Relation of shoulder to hip
- Deep core support for upper body (transversus abdominis and rectus abdominis and erector spinae strengthening)
- Side rib opening intercostal muscles

5. Elbow

- Bicep/triceps retraining
- Humerus placement
- Create spital using kinesthetic taping downward on arm

6. Wrist/hand/fingers

- Transverse carpal ligament
- Median nerve freeing
- Radial nerve freeing

Lastly, diaphragm attention: belly breathing, spinal lengthening, postural control.

I call these areas of vulnerability because that is what they are. They are vulnerable areas of the body, susceptible to extreme weakness and/or spasticity for reasons that I cannot explain other than a disconnection from the nerves, and in my opinion a disconnection from the breath, a pocket of unprocessed emotion, a kind of kink in the hose somewhere, or a blockage (physical, emotional, or mental). But by breaking through blocked areas through a consistent yoga practice, you restore the flow of oxygen into these areas of the body that may have been previously paralyzed or tight.

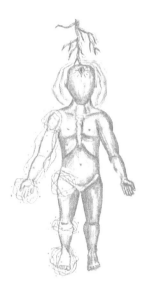

I list them in that order because they affect each other in that order, kind of like misaligning the whole leg or arm. Misalignment is a huge deal for trauma survivors, particularly stroke survivors. Getting the entire body involved in grounding poses, balancing poses, encourages this connection to reestablish and realign the body. Also, anything that lengthens the body elongates the muscles and the tendons and helps create space. Yoga is a kind of spring cleaning for the body, opening the body to other things. There is no timetable. Yoga is literally a lifelong journey. It is the ever-changing process of reuniting the mind, the body, and the spirit.

It is not one thing, it is many things, which can be very hard to understand.

But to simplify things, we translate the word yoga back to the Sanskrit word "yoke," meaning union. Union of mind, body, and Spirit. It's simple, but it works. But we cannot simplify yoga too much, for it is a *practice or a discipline*, something that takes time, patience, and consistency incorporated into everyday life. Yoga is not exercise.

The biggest thing my stroke has taught me has been to slow down. I never fully understood what that meant until I started doing yoga. But the beauty of my stroke, and I'm certain for many others, is the annoyingly beautiful way our bodies remind us to slow down. Ankle roll, shoulder subluxation, spasticity, tone, colonus, brain fog. If you have survived a stroke, you are familiar with these words. You are familiar with the way these words feel in the body.

> **Yoga is all about ALIGNMENT.**
> **Finding realignment in the body.**

They are annoying yet beautiful reminders, the body's way of beginning to reestablish communication with you. I can honestly say I have found that strokes are a way your body is saying "pay attention to me." Something was being neglected, burning the candle at both ends, forcing, rushing. They never found a medical cause for my stroke; I had none of the risk factors, not one. But I know deep down stress was the catalyst, or I should say poor stress management. Stress is a convenient excuse and, again, takes us out of ourselves. It implies that this external force is strong enough to affect our body chemistry, and I am a victim to its effects over me. Well, I don't believe that. Stress is not the enemy at all, but the more our culture makes stress the enemy, the more of an enemy it becomes. Changing your mindset on stress is something I read about in my teacher training in a book by Kelly McGonigal titled *The Upside of Stress*.

Stress is not the enemy, rather our response to stress.

Simply put, leading up to my stroke, I was running full steam ahead, like usual, and things had reached the MAX and pressure needed to go somewhere. The lid popped off, my artery burst, and a clot formed. It was bound to happen at some point; I never slowed down. I thought I was going to die, or at least be in a wheelchair watching my kids grow up from the sidelines. Strokes are not fair, and it does suck to have your life change in a split second and to all of a sudden feel like a foreigner inside yourself. I was literally in shock for the first few years. I slept the first year almost all day, every day.

I was barely surviving, getting up just to do what needed to be done before curling up back in bed while my son was in school and my infant tucked next to me. Those first few years are always the hardest. Keeping hope was very hard at times. Remember, recovery isn't a straight line or even a slope. It's more of a squiggly, mish-moshed picture a two-year-old might draw. It makes no sense to anyone but the artist and is very hard to explain.

Healing is NOT linear...
Sometimes it's downright
        MESSY!

But as I said earlier, yoga goes beyond the physical body and mind. Yoga encourages:

self-love,

self-acceptance,

self-discipline.

The three principles of *My Yoga Will*.

Three things I had no concept of prior to my stroke. Again, I put them in that order because they affect each other. You use them as stepping stones. I was never the most self-aware person. Mindfulness? Say what?

After years of teaching basic chair yoga classes in stroke survivor support groups and meeting stroke survivors so eager to do yoga, I discovered a small study done in September 2012 out of Indiana University School of Health and Rehabilitation Sciences.

To sum the study up—you can read it online anywhere—they did these poses for their eight-week study, concluding that "yoga-based rehabilitation intervention has potential in improving multiple post-stroke variables. Further testing is warranted."

2023, crickets . . .

These were the poses: "Cow, cobra, halfmoon, fish, king, and pigeon. Using 2:1 breath, mudras, eye, and head movements.

Mountain, chair locust, warrior, bridge, corpse pose, mindfulness meditation."

I have built out a similar program, teaching over 1,000 hours of yoga classes.

STROKE YOGA SEQUENCE

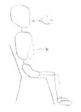
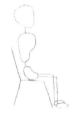
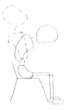

Breath Expansion
prayanama

Mountain Pose
tadasana

Spinal Flexion/ Extension
cat/cow

Child's Pose
balasana

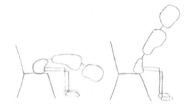
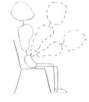

Forward Fold
uttanasana

Chair Pose
utkatasana

Sun Salutations
surya namaskar A/B

Warrior I
virabhadrasana 1

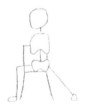
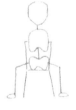

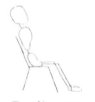

Warrior II
virabhadrasana II

Goddess
utkata konasana

Bent Knee Triangle
trikonasana

Resting Pose
savasana

CREATE YOUR OWN YOGA EXPERIENCE

CREATE YOUR OWN YOGA EXPERIENCE

CREATE YOUR OWN YOGA EXPERIENCE

Duration/Notes	Description
seated 1–4 weeks	**soft hum** *chanting OHM SATYA OHM* mouth scrunching/lip pursing head and neck movements-side to side breathwork foundation firm grounding through feet activating hamstrings notice length and rise through the spine mental awareness to feet, relaxing lifting the toes/curling toes lifting heels, stretching bottom of foot dorsiflexion/plantar flexion shoulder rolls extension/flexion of head and neck hip hinge, coming to standing with balance bar or back of chair, slowly Breath expansion Mountain pose Cat cow Child's pose Forward fold Chair pose Sun sals Warrior 1 Warrior II Goddess bent one triangle Resting pose

Savasana with yoga nidra

Add ins:
Preparation cobbler pose, bound angle (Supta badha) with second chair or staff pose (Dandasana)

Mudra weeks 1–4:
Namaskar (linga) Mudra: interlock prayer pose, hands at heart, finger counting both hands,* brain connections
Gyana mudra: index and thumb join *concentration
dhyana mudra: thumbs join
*promotes patience and stability

Mantra weeks 1–4:
I am present within my body.
I can center my body with the ease of my breath.
I am confident, grounded, worthy, and whole.
I am here now.
Side Plank (Utthita Vasisthasana)

Duration/Notes	Description
standing	standing with eyes closed holding bar or chair
4–6 weeks	pronation/supination of wrist
	shoulder blades up and back down
	step back
	Yin-style holds with three-part breath or Ujjayi(depending on client BP)
	breath holds: squeezing up face/hands, holding breath
	and releasing. Repeat
	Vinyasa-type flow moving
	possibility for arms to reach over head, halfway
	lift and forward bend
	down to floor if accessible
	lowering down to floor onto knees, balancing on knees
	Warrior 1 (Virabhadrasana)
	Crescent lunge on knee (Anjaneyasana)
	Warrior 2 (Trikonasana) in chair
	Bent knee triangle
	Side plank in chair
	Sun salutations A
	Camel pose (Ushtrasana)
	Cobbler pose with bolster

Add-ins:
Triangle and revolved triangle
(Trikonasana)
Sun salutations A
Camel pose (Ushtrasana)
Child's pose (Balasana)
Hero pose (Virasana)
modified side plank, optional
cobbler pose (Supta Baddha Konasana)
Modified pigeon pose (kapotasana)
Balancing tree at wall
Savasana final resting (Savasana)
Yoga Nidra, optional

Mudras week 4–6
Shambhala Mudra: one hand in fist
opposite hand over it
**promotes positive thinking
Adi mudra: fold in thumb and make fist
**stimulates blood flow

Mantra week 4–6
"Breathing in, I calm my body.
Breathing out, I smile.
Dwelling in the present moment.
I know this is a wonderful moment."
~Ancient Native Mantra
SO HUM: inhale/exhale
**I AM

What did you feel after your first yoga class?

....
....
....
....
....
....
....
....
....
....
....
....
....
....
....
....
....
....
....
....
....
....
....
....
....
....

READING/REFERENCE LIST

The Power of Now by Eckhart Tolle

Autobiography of a Yogi by Paramahyna Yogananda

A New Earth by Eckhart Tolle

The Yoga Sutras of Patanjali, translation by Swami Satchadinanda

The Upside of Stress by Kelly McGonigal, PhD

How Yoga Works by Geshe Michael Roach

Meditation and its Practice by Swami Rama

The Journey Within by Radhanath

Be Here Now by Ram Dass

Any Westerner's translation of *The Bhagavad Gita*

Breathing the Master Key to Self Healing by Dr. Andrew Weil

CHAPTER 14

CHAKRA JOURNALING

1. Do you feel you have purpose in your life? Explain any connection to the divine. Do you connect with the divine within?

....
....
....
....
....
....

2. When is the earliest age you remember having a gut feeling?
Define intuition. Were you encouraged to trust yourself?

....
....
....
....
....
....

3. Is there anything you'd like the world to hear you say?

Have you been speaking your truth? Too much or too little?

Create an inner dialogue with you now and eleven-year-old you. What would you say to her or him? What do you think he or she would say to you?

What was communication like at home?

………………………………………………………………………
………………………………………………………………………
………………………………………………………………………
………………………………………………………………………
………………………………………………………………………
………………………………………………………………………
………………………………………………………………………

4. When you look around, what breaks your heart? Are you open to receiving love? How would you define compassion, and what does it mean to you to show compassion?

………………………………………………………………………
………………………………………………………………………
………………………………………………………………………
………………………………………………………………………
………………………………………………………………………
………………………………………………………………………
………………………………………………………………………
………………………………………………………………………

5. Do your personal habits support who you want to be in the world?

Who do you want to be in this world? Change "have tos" to "want tos." Think action and purpose.

....
....
....
....
....
....
....
....
....

6. Are you stimulating your creative passions? What is something you'd like to try? What will you bring to 2024?

....
....
....
....
....
....
....
....

7. **What do I need in my life to feel more grounded and secure? Think early childhood. How do you nourish yourself?**

....

....

....

....

....

....

....

....

....

....

....

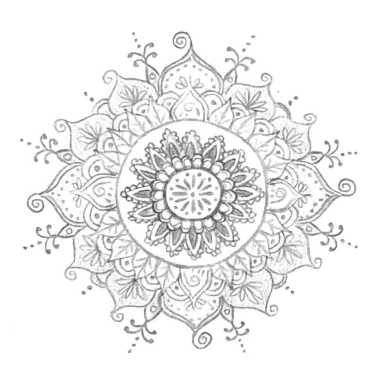

Subtle Stroke

Subtle Stroke

Rachel Jarmusz

Rachel Jarmusz

Rachel Jarmusz

Rachel Jarmusz

Rachel Jarmusz

....
....
....
....
....
....
....
....
....
....
....
....
....
....
....
....
....
....
....
....
....
....
....
....

Rachel Jarmusz

....
....
....
....
....
....
....
....
....
....
....
....
....
....
....
....
....
....
....
....
....
....
....

Rachel Jarmusz

....
....
....
....
....
....
....
....
....
....
....
....
....
....
....
....
....
....
....
....
....
....
....
....
....

Rachel Jarmusz

....
....
....
....
....
....
....
....
....
....
....
....
....
....
....
....
....
....
....
....
....
....
....
....
....

....
....
....
....
....
....
....
....
....
....
....
....
....
....
....
....
....
....
....
....
....
....
....
....
....
....

Subtle Stroke

Rachel Jarmusz

....
....
....
....
....
....
....
....
....
....
....
....
....
....
....
....
....
....
....
....
....
....
....
....
....
....

....
....
....
....
....
....
....
....
....
....
....
....
....
....
....
....
....
....
....
....
....
....
....
....
....

....
....
....
....
....
....
....
....
....
....
....
....
....
....
....
....
....
....
....
....
....
....
....
....
....

Subtle Stroke

Rachel Jarmusz

....
....
....
....
....
....
....
....
....
....
....
....
....
....
....
....
....
....
....
....
....
....
....
....
....
....

Rachel Jarmusz

....
....
....
....
....
....
....
....
....
....
....
....
....
....
....
....
....
....
....
....
....
....
....
....
....

Rachel Jarmusz

....
....
....
....
....
....
....
....
....
....
....
....
....
....
....
....
....
....
....
....
....
....
....
....
....

....
....
....
....
....
....
....
....
....
....
....
....
....
....
....
....
....
....
....
....
....
....
....
....
....

Rachel Jarmusz

....
....
....
....
....
....
....
....
....
....
....
....
....
....
....
....
....
....
....
....
....
....
....
....
....

Rachel Jarmusz

Rachel Jarmusz

Rachel Jarmusz

....
....
....
....
....
....
....
....
....
....
....
....
....
....
....
....
....
....
....
....
....
....
....
....

....
....
....
....
....
....
....
....
....
....
....
....
....
....
....
....
....
....
....
....
....
....
....
....
....
....

Rachel Jarmusz

Subtle Stroke

Rachel Jarmusz

....
....
....
....
....
....
....
....
....
....
....
....
....
....
....
....
....
....
....
....
....
....
....
....

Rachel Jarmusz

Rachel Jarmusz

Rachel Jarmusz

....
....
....
....
....
....
....
....
....
....
....
....
....
....
....
....
....
....
....
....
....
....
....
....

Rachel Jarmusz

....
....
....
....
....
....
....
....
....
....
....
....
....
....
....
....
....
....
....
....
....
....
....
....
....

Subtle Stroke

Rachel Jarmusz

....
....
....
....
....
....
....
....
....
....
....
....
....
....
....
....
....
....
....
....
....
....
....
....
....

Rachel Jarmusz

....
....
....
....
....
....
....
....
....
....
....
....
....
....
....
....
....
....
....
....
....
....
....
....
....

Subtle Stroke

Rachel Jarmusz

....
....
....
....
....
....
....
....
....
....
....
....
....
....
....
....
....
....
....
....
....
....
....
....
....
....

Rachel Jarmusz

....
....
....
....
....
....
....
....
....
....
....
....
....
....
....
....
....
....
....
....
....
....
....
....
....
....

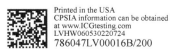